CONSTANT
CRAVING

D0973987

CONSTANT CRAVING

*What Your Food Cravings Mean
and How to Overcome Them*

Doreen Virtue

HAY HOUSE, INC.
Carlsbad, California • New York City
London • Sydney • Johannesburg
Vancouver • Hong Kong • New Delhi

Published and distributed in the United States by: Hay House, Inc.

Editorial supervision: Jill Kramer
Cover design: Amy Rose Grigoriou

ISBN: 978-1-4019-3549-8

In loving memory of
my grandmother,
Pearl E. Reynolds

C O N T E N T S

Constant Craving brings together many years of scientific, psychological, and metaphysical research about food cravings. I wrote this book so you, the reader, can interpret and control your emotionally based overeating. This is a book for anyone who wants to lose weight and maintain that weight loss through the natural process of appetite reduction.

My education about weight and appetite stems from first-hand experience with food cravings. I've learned that maintaining weight loss hinges upon maintaining peace of mind. I've also worked with countless women and men around the globe, helping them naturally reduce their food cravings.

I first became interested in the study of appetite as a result of my own struggles with cravings for ice cream and bread. As the daughter of a mother who was a Christian Science practitioner, and a father who wrote and edited books about not accepting any limitations, I was raised to believe that we are born perfect, in the image and likeness of our Creator, and that physical and mental problems stem from psychological sources. I grew up with the understanding that false beliefs, unloving thoughts, and fear-based expectations breed illness, accidents, and disease.

So, when my own appetite went out of control in my early 20s, I naturally searched for its emotional roots. At that time, there were no eating-disorder books or support groups. I had to search for my own answers to uncover my compulsion to binge-eat ice cream and bread.

It is said that when the student is ready, the teacher will appear. Well, my teacher appeared as I worked as a drug abuse and alcoholism counselor at a hospital. As you'll read in Chapter 1, I discovered that each of my clients' personality styles corresponded to his or her drug of choice. Those addicted to heroin were very different from those addicted to marijuana, and alcoholics had personalities that were entirely different from cocaine abusers. On and on, I catalogued the personality and drug-of-choice correlations.

I thought I was researching *other* people, but little did I know I was researching my own self! My revelation hit me when I was working with several heroin addicts. I'd never gone near the drug, never seen it, and had no inkling what a heroin craving felt like. To be able to empathize with the addicts' descriptions of heroin cravings, I had to think about my own yearnings for chocolate cake and ice cream. The addicts would describe feeling helplessly drawn toward a syringe, and I would mentally replace the image of heroin with an image of chocolate cake. Through this process, I was able to more accurately relate to my clients' cravings.

In the beginning, I have to admit that at some level I was judging these heroin addicts. Well, what a hypocrite I was being! Here *they* were, voluntarily getting counseling and treatment, while every evening I would waltz out of the hospital unit and head straight to the nearest Baskin-Robbins ice cream shop! The moment I confronted myself honestly—*your patients are getting help for their addictions, while you are still wallowing in your food addiction*—there was no turning back. I had no choice but to get well.

The next 11 years produced so much healing, knowledge, and realized dreams. I came to understand why I was so hungry all the time: I was afraid of my gut feelings. My gut was telling me to make changes in my marriage and career, and I was afraid to trust what it was saying. I thought I'd fail! So I poured food on my gut to suppress its voice.

When I finally listened to my gut instead of smothering it with food, my life radically shifted. I transformed myself from a fat, unhappy woman with little money or romance in her life, into a trim-figured psychotherapist rich in friendship, love, and financial success. I learned that our gut never fails us; it is *we* who fail to heed its wisdom and trust its guidance.

After that, I devoted myself to studying eating disorders and the psychological issues triggering food cravings. I found that, as was the case with my drug-addicted clients, each food craving corresponds to a particular personality style and emotional issue. I began sharing my food-craving interpretations with workshop audiences and clients, with remarkable results. Because, instead of spending hours, days, or months uncovering an emotional issue, I found that the use of food-craving interpretations allowed me to bypass my clients' defense mechanisms and go straight to the heart of the matter.

The result of all my research is now in your hands. Here is the information you need to really get honest with yourself about *why* you are craving certain foods. I've also packed in lots of suggestions and helpful advice about ways to prevent eating binges, reduce emotional eating, and regain a balanced appetite.

The journey from overeating to normal eating isn't simple, but it is a necessity. To me, it's a choice between imprisonment in a "fat cell," and freedom in a carefree spirit and light body. I hope that, as I did, you'll choose to break free from your fat cell!

— Doreen Virtue
  Hawaii

A C K N O W L E D G M E N T S

I want to thank Jill Kramer, Reid Tracy, Kristina Tracy, Jeannie Liberati, Christy Salinas, Amy Rose Grigoriou, Bill and Joan Hannan, Ada Montgomery, Pearl E. Reynolds, Mary Baker Eddy, Catherine Ponder, Forest Holly, Marianne Williamson, Norman Vincent Peale, Sheldon Kopp, Viktor Frankl, Grant Virtue, and Chuck Virtue.

Deep gratitude to my clients, workshop audiences, and the many women who wrote to me after reading my first Hay House book, *Losing Your Pounds of Pain: Breaking the Link Between Abuse, Stress, and Overeating*. Your openness in expressing your frustrations and hopes has touched me like nothing else. Thank you so much for responding to the book's true message of healing!

TRUST YOUR GUT FEELINGS

Note: *Throughout this book, I've used numerical footnotes [1] whenever I'm discussing another researcher's material. They correspond to the numbered "Notes" listings in the Appendix of the book. The footnotes do not contain any additional material; they are a reference if you want to read further about a particular topic. If you choose to disregard the footnote numbers as you're reading, you won't miss any of the meaning or message in this book.*

INTRODUCTION:
FAT IS A SPIRITUAL ISSUE

Every part of you is perfect, whole, and complete; and your appetite is no exception. Your food cravings and voracious appetite don't mean that something is wrong with you or that you are weak in any way. Rather, they show that your appetite is operating *exactly* as intended.

Your entire body, including your appetite, reflects the level of peace of mind in your life. Your appetite is designed like an airplane instrument panel—to warn you when spiritual and emotional fuel run low. Hunger is a flashing red light signaling, "I need more peace of mind!"

Animals put on extra weight in preparation for winter hibernation. Humans who carry extra weight are in a spiritual hibernation, asleep to their true potential. The weight serves as a hedge against perceived dangers and lack, in a world that, in truth, is filled with safety and abundance. It's time to wake up from the heavy, tired hibernation of overweight and overeating. When you walk out of the dark winter cave and into the daylight, you experience your true state of eternal springtime, filled with creativity, success, and energy!

In the past, you may have tried to *kill* your appetite with external forces such as diets, powders, or pills. As you discovered, that approach didn't work for long. What is needed, instead, is to *heal* your appetite using an internal approach. Well, that's exactly the approach you will be offered in these pages.

It's no accident that you crave a particular food at a particular moment. We crave foods that we hope will give us peace of mind. Cravings occur for two reasons: a desire to feel better emotionally, or to shift our energy level. We want to feel peppier or calmer. More secure and confident. Less angry. Or less afraid.

All creatures are driven to fulfill their basic needs for food, water, rest, shelter, and peace of mind. If any of these needs go unfulfilled, your body signals you to correct the situation. This process of maintaining a comfortable, healthy balance in your body and mind is called *homeostasis*.

The homeostatic drive tells you to put on a jacket when you're cold, drink when you're thirsty, and sleep when you're tired. When you lose peace of mind, your gut feelings direct you to take action to correct the troubling situation. If you don't take action, you experience a negative emotion such as depression. Still, your body is driven to maintain homeostasis, so it tries another approach with you. Your appetite knows which foods will deliver your desired emotion or energy level—those that will bring you back to a temporary state of peace of mind.

Every food you crave has mood- or energy-altering properties that will return you to a temporary homeostasis. As you'll read further on, your body's natural intelligence is remarkable.

Gut Feelings

Our gut is the center of our emotions. We feel fear, excitement, anger, and love in our midsection. You've probably had one of these experiences:

+ You had butterflies of excitement in your stomach.
+ You were newly in love, and lost your appetite as a result.
+ Your intuition came in the form of a "gut feeling."

+ You got knots in your stomach, when you felt anxious or afraid.
+ You had nausea or a stomachache when you were nervous.
+ You felt hungry because you were lonely, bored, or stressed.
+ You were worried sick.
+ You couldn't "swallow" or "stomach" an unpleasant situation.
+ Someone tried to "feed" you a pack of lies.
+ You were hungry for attention or love.
+ You were "fed"-up with someone.

Our intuition, or gut feelings, directs and guides us. Our gut is the link between the intelligence of the universe and our human experience. This inner voice encompasses a million years of wisdom inherited from our cave-dwelling ancestors. It tells us whether or not a person is acting honorably, which career path to take, what house to buy, which person to marry, and so on.

When we listen to our gut feelings, we're always rewarded with peace of mind. When our gut's instructions seem frightening ("I'm too scared to pursue the career of my dreams because I'm afraid of failing!"), we muffle the volume of our inner voice by pouring substances into our gut, such as food or alcohol.

I was 22 years old when I first experienced this phenomenon. I was a young mother in an emotionally and financially impoverished marriage. My husband and I were struggling to pay the rent and feed our sons. We'd fight all the time due to our stress and fear. And every day, the mailman brought a steady stream of overdue bill notices.

My husband was the human embodiment of fear, and one of his overriding worries was that I would leave him for another man. To combat this fear, he fed me a steady diet of negative talk. He told me I was fat, ugly, stupid, worthless, and that no other man would want me—especially since I had two children. He told the lie so often that I eventually believed it. His lies hypnotized me and convinced me that I did not deserve better.

Still, I kept seeing this inner vision of the life I was supposed to have. Like a slide show in my mind, I saw images of myself as a light, free spirit. In my wide-awake dream, I envisioned myself as a psychotherapist and author, living in a house next to the water, with a healthy, fit, trim body. I know now that this was God speaking to me through my gut feelings.

Whenever I allowed myself to acknowledge this dream, I would feel overwhelming intimidation! I shared my dream with my husband, and suffered his ridicule. How could I, an uneducated housewife with family responsibilities, no money, and a complete lack of self-confidence, even imagine the realization of such a lofty goal? That inner vision scared me because I didn't believe I deserved good. Other people deserved good, but not me. In that way, my gut feelings triggered fear in me.

The direct way to deal with this type of fear is to trust your gut instincts and follow their direction. But at first, I chose the unproductive alternative of silencing my gut feelings by overeating. I poured food on my gut, got fatter, and used this fatness as additional confirmation that I was unworthy of achieving my goals.

In time, I was sufficiently humbled by my failures and life pain to admit, "I don't know what I'm doing!" When I finally let go and allowed God to take over, I started trusting my gut feelings. I listened to this inner source of direction and allowed myself to believe in it. I trusted that God would not have given me a mission without also backing it up with sufficient supplies of talent, creativity, and courage.

That was the best decision I ever made. I have come to understand that every time my life goes astray, it's because I'm not listening to my inner voice. That's when I lose my peace of mind, and as a result, I experience intense food cravings. Then I overeat, and it becomes a vicious cycle.

But when I began listening to my inner voice, I was given the direction to fulfill my dreams. I took college courses, wrote manuscripts, and maintained a clear and focused vision of my dreams. My gut feelings guided me through setbacks and challenges. With hard work and prayer, I became the person whom I had envisioned so many times—a psychotherapist and bestselling author who regularly appears on national television.

All my needs and wants are taken care of, because I know now that I deserve good. You deserve good, too. We all deserve good.

We can't go wrong when we follow our gut. We fulfill our Divine purpose, which ultimately helps other people, especially our family members. We have no reason to overeat when our mind is settled and at peace. Following your gut creates miracles in your life!

Time to Heal

If you've struggled with weight and dieting, then you already know how to lose weight better than anyone! Eat less fat and exercise more—it's not rocket science. Yet, the reason why Americans are heavier than ever is due to our overactive appetites. *If we weren't hungry all the time, there would be no weight problems.*

The material in this book will help you reduce the power of your food cravings. By interpreting *why* you are craving a particular food, your cravings will dissipate or disappear. You'll feel more in control of your food choices. Instead of that box of cookies commanding you to eat, you'll feel free to eat one, two, or no cookies at all.

You are about to learn my little-known method of food-craving interpretation. Once you know how to interpret your food cravings, your urges to overeat will never overwhelm you again.

The Nightmare of Food Cravings

Food-craving interpretation is similar to the interpretation of bad dreams. After all, nightmares and food cravings share a lot in common. We have bad dreams whenever we avoid facing uncomfortable thoughts or feelings. Food cravings also signal unresolved emotions.

The two methods of dealing with nightmares and food cravings are identical. In the first method, you directly address the source of your upset about work, finances, friends, love, family, health, or whatever. Sometimes, though, the cause of the upheaval isn't readily apparent. Often, we're not ready to face the truth about our conflicting feelings and beliefs. Those fears block us from making changes that yield peace of mind.

In those cases, the most practical route is to *interpret* the bad dream or food craving. Interpretation holds a mirror up to your face, enabling you to instantly recognize the true source of your emotional discomfort or pain. Once you uncover the source, you take the appropriate action and then *let go* of the past.

Dream interpretation has been studied since Freud's time, and most therapists such as myself regularly include this therapeutic practice within the course of treatment. It helps the therapist and the client bypass defenses and quickly understand the deep-seated beliefs triggering unhealthful behavior.

Years ago, when I began interpreting food cravings, I found that these interpretations were much more reliable than those related to dreams, because fewer variables exist. In dream interpretation, the therapist must gauge what the various symbols mean to the dreamer. Water, colors, buildings, vehicles, and people are common dream symbols that hold completely different meanings and significance depending on the individual.

With food cravings, though, the meanings behind each food are much more consistent. For example, interpreting what a craving for crunchy peanut butter means remains constant; this type of craving almost always signifies a person who is stressed, angry, or frustrated and who is in need of some fun and recreation.

Every food corresponds to a certain mood. Any time your appetite goes out of control, it's because you want to feel more energetic, more relaxed, or in a better mood. Intuitively, your cravings are for the exact food that will produce the desired effect.

Others, besides me, have studied the relationship between mood and food cravings. Their studies back up my conclusions that you can accurately assess an emotional issue just by knowing what food is being craved.

For example, Bernard Lyman, Ph.D., a university professor from British Columbia, asked 200 subjects to imagine themselves experiencing 22 different emotions, including anger, boredom, depression, loneliness, and joy. While the study participants imagined themselves experiencing each emotion, Dr. Lyman asked them what food they'd like to eat.

The results were statistically significant—in other words, more meaningful than you'd expect to see just by chance. Specific food preferences consistently corresponded to each of the emotions. The table on the following page illustrates some of Dr. Lyman's findings. I find it interesting that "anxiety" produced such a strong craving for snacks—both the healthy type and the "junky" variety—and that "love" and "happiness" triggered strong preferences for dessert (probably chocolate, although this study didn't make that distinction). On the basis of his research, Dr. Lyman concluded, "Different preferences clearly go with different emotions."[1]

Percentage of 200 Students Reporting Food Cravings in Response to Elicited Emotions

	Anxious	Happy	Loving	Self-Confident	Solemn
Salad	2	5	12	11	6
Soup	6	1	0	2	6
Eggs	3	1	2	3	1
Fish	0	4	4	15	3
Meat	11	29	28	26	23
Poultry	0	3	1	6	5
Casseroles	2	6	2	8	3
Fast Foods	6	12	6	4	2
Vegetables	3	23	16	11	18
Cheese	1	6	4	6	0
Fruit	6	11	10	7	7
Sandwiches	8	4	2	3	3
Dessert	3	15	10	1	3
Milk	5	2	1	0	2
Juice	2	1	0	1	0
Healthy Snacks	20	13	9	7	8
Junk Snacks	22	9	7	1	3
Non-Alcoholic					
drinks	11	6	3	6	8
Alcohol	0	6	14	3	0
Nothing	19	3	18	7	17
Anything	4	8	12	14	5
Not Sure	2	3	6	3	9

Source: Lyman, 1982[1]

Heal Your Appetite, Don't Kill Your Appetite

I think you'll enjoy learning about food-craving interpretation. When I give speeches and talk-show appearances on the subject of food cravings, audience members always want their food cravings interpreted. I decided to write this book so you could learn how to conduct your own interpretations, as well as interpret your friends' and family's food cravings.

You'll be amazed by the wisdom of your appetite, and by how accurate your intuition is with respect to craving the exact food that corresponds to your desired emotional or energy state!

Let me ask you: when it comes to your appetite, eating habits, or weight, do your food cravings seem to control you? Do you sometimes feel you have no choice but to eat the food you are craving? Are there times when all you can think about is food? Whether you crave chocolate, cheeseburgers, bread, or ice cream, isn't it the height of frustration to struggle with food cravings?!

Your stomach says, "I want to eat it—NOW!"

To which your mind counters, "No, you can't eat it. It's fattening. You need to lose weight. Forget about that food."

However, your stomach replies, "But I want it!" The more your mind says no, the more you want to eat it.

We all know, deep down, that our hunger is rarely physically based. Our hunger is usually a desire to feel better *right now*. Like a caged animal pacing to and fro, your appetite circles around all your thoughts, plans, and energy. You imagine details about the food you crave: what it tastes like, where to buy it, how to prepare it. You imagine, too, how you'll "undo" the calories and fat grams by skipping breakfast or exercising.

It's an addictive cycle, where the pursuit of food takes over much of your life. Suddenly, you are no longer in control. Food is. But, if you're like me, you don't want to fight yourself the rest of your life. The good news is that you don't have to. Weight and eating issues don't have to represent a continual struggle between will power and appetite when you:

Turn your focus away from maintaining a weight loss, and instead turn your focus to maintaining peace of mind.

As long as you maintain peace of mind, your appetite will never feel out of control again! But sometimes, it's confusing to know exactly what will deliver you from the turmoil and give you this peace. That's where food-craving interpretation can help you—by letting you know which area of your life needs attention.

Every food you crave corresponds to a specific emotion or issue calling for your attention. When you're depressed, you're likely to crave a dairy product such as cheese or ice cream. When you're anxious, you'll go for something crunchy such as chips or nuts. In fact, there's a biological and psychological reason for each and every food you crave. Once you uncover the underlying emotion, you'll feel a sense of relief stemming from being honest with yourself. At that point, your craving will diminish.

Every food contains minerals, amino acids, textures, smells, and other mood- and energy-influencing properties. Some are stimulants, some are depressants, and some activate the pleasure centers in our brains. In fact, many food's mood-altering or "psychoactive" properties are identical to those found in prescription medications for depression, anxiety, and asthma!

The mood you intuitively wish to experience determines which food you'll crave. For example, if you feel depressed or lethargic, you will crave foods that brighten your mood. If you feel tense or irritable, you'll crave foods that will soothe your nerves. Feeling bored? Your cravings will steer you toward foods that trigger pleasure- or excitement-inducing chemicals in your brain.

To back up these types of findings, I've included material in this book that is based on extensive research from three sources:

1. *Scientific studies,* from universities around the world, about the psychoactive (mood-altering) properties of various foods. In addition, I've compiled the latest studies about appetite in animals, human infants, and human adults; food preferences, and the effect of exercise on neurochemicals and appetite.

2. *Ancient Chinese medicine* theories about the "energies" of food. Amazingly, Chinese beliefs about food's stimulating and calming properties dovetail perfectly with modern scientific research! The foods that were labeled "hot" (the Chinese medicine description of a stimulant, not the flavor) centuries ago, are the very foods that today are called vasoconstrictors, or stimulants.

3. *One-on-one interviews,* conducted in clinical sessions and at my workshops. By studying thousands of women and men, I was able to correlate their food cravings to their emotional issues and mood preferences. I also kept detailed records of my own food cravings and corresponding moods.

Amazingly, all three of these information sources—modern scientific research, ancient Chinese medicine beliefs, and my personal interviews—draw similar conclusions about which foods correspond to which emotions.

Food Cravings Are Key

Everyone gets hungry, of course. But beyond *normal* appetite, and way beyond Thanksgiving eating binges, are overwhelming food cravings that are incessant, annoying, and invasive. What's more, these food cravings destroy well-intentioned nutrition and dieting plans.

Here's how I define a *food craving*: *An obsessive desire for a specific type of food.* This is different from just feeling hungry for anything that happens to be in the fridge or cupboard. It's also different from overeating, say, peanuts or popcorn, just because they happen to be available. Food cravings are specific thoughts and desires for a certain type or category of food, such as chocolate, potato chips, or Mexican food. Occasionally, a "healthful" craving for fruit, vegetables, or whole grains comes up, but most cravings are for high-fat, highly processed foods.

Whereas having a normal, healthy appetite, with moderate eating habits, is pleasurable, obsessive food cravings are annoying. Cravings interfere with our freedom to choose between eating, and abstaining from, food. Cravings control us, and nobody enjoys being controlled.

This I firmly believe: *Overwhelming food cravings are the culprit behind every obese body, every broken diet, and every dietary-related disease.* If we can stop the food cravings, the unhealthful eating habits will disappear. After all, obesity is not caused by a lack of nutritional knowledge, but an overactive appetite. If we weren't hungry so much of the time, we'd have no reason to overeat, would we?

At one time in our culture, we could blame public ignorance for this country's unhealthful eating habits. But today, most people have heard recommendations for a balanced, low-fat diet in conjunction with regular exercise. Practically every school child learns basic nutrition, and anyone with media access—magazines, newspapers, radio, or television—has heard the dietary drumbeat to eat more fruits and vegetables, and cut down on saturated fat. This information surrounds us!

Two studies revealed the extent of dietary knowledge possessed by the average person. In 1958, researchers asked 300 British women about the nutritional makeup of foods. Twenty years later, another group of researchers asked a similar group of 300 women the same questions. Look at the difference 20 years can make![2]

Percentage of Awareness of Food Components Among a Sample of 300 Women

	1958	**1978**
Vitamins	44%	98%
Protein	27%	97%
Calories	14%	96%
Carbohydrates	3%	86%
Fat	3%	94%

Sources: Jenkins; British Nutrition Foundation[2]

If the same survey were conducted today, the amount of nutritional awareness would probably be even closer to 100 percent. Yet, Americans are heavier than ever—34 percent are clinically overweight, compared to 25 percent in 1988, according to the National Center for Health Statistics. Why is this the case at a time when almost anyone who has read a health book, a magazine, or talked with a physician, knows the importance of a low-fat diet and regular exercise? I believe that emotional overeating is the culprit behind the expanding American beltline.

Lack of nutritional information is clearly not the problem. One study actually found that obese and dieting people were significantly more knowledgeable about nutrition than normal-weight and non-dieting people.[3] Nutritionist Jane Thomas studied the relationship between nutritional knowledge and food choices and concluded, "...it seems clear that food practices do not change just because people are in possession of accurate factual knowledge."[4]

Although fat consumption is down in the average American household, the total number of calories we eat has risen. As the stress and uncertainty in our lives increases, we naturally seek a source of comfort and solace. For many people, that source is food.

Only one type of knowledge leads to healthier eating: an understanding of *why* you are craving a certain type of food. Once you acknowledge that your cravings for peanut butter cookies or some other food actually mean that you are craving comfort and fun, your appetite won't seem so overwhelming and utterly controlling.

What's Weight Got to Do with It?

I have worked with compulsive overeaters for many years, and I have always been impressed by their sophisticated knowledge of nutrition. Each of my clients (mostly female) could recite the approximate caloric, fat, and carbohydrate content of practically any food you could name. They owned dozens of diet books and had read many magazine weight-loss articles. Every client knew *how* to lose weight—as I've said, a lack of dietary knowledge is not the problem. The actual problem was their appetite, which was completely out of control. Like a horse with the bit in his mouth whose rider helplessly hangs on for dear life, these clients had appetites that had completely taken over.

It didn't matter how many diet books or magazine articles, how many gym memberships or how many size-7 jeans they'd buy for "motivation," my clients' weight was always determined by the magnitude of their food cravings.

These are some of the comments that I have heard most frequently:

> "How can I get rid of my urges to eat chocolate?"
> "Help! I can't stop eating french fries and cheeseburgers! I know they're fattening, but my cravings are overwhelming. What can I do?"
> "Why do I crave ice cream all the time?"
> "All I seem to want to do is snack on crunchy, salty things night and day!"

Isn't it maddening to have this one area of your life—eating—so out of your control?

Let me emphasize that I am not advocating dieting. I'd be the first person celebrating in the streets if our culture would loosen some of its rigid standards about weight. If people choose to have overweight bodies, and *really* believe that they are happy—fine. As long as they feel great about the amount of food they are eating and their energy levels, there's no problem. But if these people are truly honest, they will probably admit that food cravings bug them a little. Okay, they bug them a lot! After all, nobody enjoys being controlled.

When I carried 50 extra pounds of fat on my body, I desperately wanted to believe that I was happy. I'd sit in front of the TV eating ice cream straight from the carton, thinking that I was in heaven. But I was actually pouring ice cream on top of my gut feelings that told me, "You're not living the life you are supposed to be living!" I didn't want to look at how disfigured my life had become.

As I've previously mentioned, I was a fat, unhappy housewife who was selling herself short. I had a dream, deep inside of me, to be a professional success, living in the home of my dreams. But that dream scared me to death! I was so afraid of failure that I tried to drown my awareness of these goals. As long as I kept my stomach full, I could pretend that my life was just fine. Instead of trusting my gut, I poured food on it.

Well, that method only made my life get worse and my body get fatter. I was deeply in debt, in constant fights with my husband, and insecure about my intelligence, self-worth, and attractiveness. As bad as my life felt, I feared that if I made any changes, my life would worsen. The more I ignored my gut feelings, the more intense my food cravings became. How ironic it all seems, looking back. The answers were always there—those that would heal my dismal life as well as my weight problems.

Once I was sufficiently humbled by life pain, I let go of trying to control everyone and everything. Out of desperation, I began listening to the inner voice in my gut, which helped put me on the right path.

It's a daily balancing act, this listening to the gut. Every time I obey its instructions, I am bathed in peace of mind and there are no food cravings. When I ignore my inner voice and try to control things, I lose my peace of mind and food cravings reappear. I use food-craving analysis on myself at that point as a direct pipeline to my gut's conversation.

If we didn't have the compulsion to overeat, there would be no weight problems. If our food cravings stayed at normal levels, we would never be tempted to finish an entire package of potato chips, carton of ice cream, or canister of nuts. This point bears repeating: *We only overeat because some haunting feeling compels us to eat, in the hope that the food will make us feel better, happier, and more energetic.*

So, if you're sick of having your food cravings bully you around, great! Let's do something about it. Read on, and you'll find out why your emotions and energy levels drive you to binge-eat. You'll also read about alternatives to overeating that will give you the emotional relief you are seeking.

Instead of trying to *kill* your appetite, you can *heal* your appetite!

Your Cravings Mean Something

I began my psychotherapy career as an alcohol and drug abuse counselor at a CareUnit hospital in Southern California. It was quite an education. I spent a great deal of time talking with the patients, and noticed that each drug abuser's drug of choice seemed predetermined by their personalities and emotional issues—that is, cocaine abusers were quite different from those who smoked marijuana to excess.

Even the patients hooked on multiple drug combinations had unique personalities. The cocaine addicts tended to seesaw between workaholic and devil-may-care lifestyles. They were driven to action, both by their personalities and by their drug of choice. Then they slept (for days!) or shirked all responsibilities.

The marijuana addicts, in contrast, had intense fears of being "hyperactive," and used pot to slow themselves down. The drug created mood swings, though—when they "came down," marijuana addicts displayed some of the grouchiest temperaments I had ever seen. When they lit up a joint, however, their spirits correspondingly lightened up as well.

The more cases I worked on, the more the clear distinctions in personality styles between different drug users fascinated me.

After a couple of years working with addicts and alcoholics, I had the opportunity to open and direct an eating-disorder program. I was startled to discover that these clients also had remarkable personality differences, which seemed contingent upon the foods they most often ate.

People who binged on chocolate were unlike those who binged on cheeseburgers. And those clients who overate dairy products were very different from those who craved bread.

It wasn't long before I could discern a person's emotional issues just by hearing what food they craved. In 1990, I began appearing on national and regional talk shows and giving lectures on the topic of food cravings. Every time someone would tell me their food craving, I was always able to pinpoint the underlying cause. I even accurately interpreted the food cravings of Phil Donahue, Geraldo Rivera, and Sally Jessy Raphael on live national television (this was really sticking my neck out, in the firm belief that my theories were correct).

I began researching appetite and food cravings, and was startled to discover how many psychoactive food ingredients were identical to prescription and illegal drug ingredients! For example, *phenylethylamine,* in chocolate, is the primary ingredient in an illegal "designer drug" called *Ecstasy*, formerly known as MDMA. *Tyramine* and *pyrazine*, ingredients in nuts, coffee, pickled foods, sour cream, aged cheese, and other foods, are the basis of antidepressant medications and asthma bronchia-dilators.

No wonder there were so many correlations between food cravings and my experiences with addicts! Food cravings were a mirror image of the prescription and illegal drug cravings I'd witnessed at the hospital years before. The only difference was that overindulgence in food lacked the moral, social, and legal ramifications of drug abuse. I also concluded that drug addicts have an easier time "kicking the habit" than food addicts. After all, you can live without drugs, but not without food. Every day, we are faced with decisions and choices about what foods to eat, and which to avoid.

The Natural Approach to Weight Loss

We do ourselves a huge disfavor when we try to kill our appetite with herbs, "dieter's teas," or pills. Our food cravings are a source of emotional education! Instead of trying to *kill* our appetite, we can *heal* our appetite by listening to its wisdom.

This is the natural approach to weight loss. We were meant to be light in spirit and body, not dragged down with worry, depression, frustration, or guilt! Once we interpret our food cravings and understand their true meaning, the appetite naturally normalizes. When the appetite reduces, you naturally eat less food. Weight loss always follows.

If this sounds simple, it's because it is! That's the beauty of this approach to eating and weight loss. Instead of fighting yourself, instead of struggling against your natural urges, you'll be "letting go." Your old methods of fighting your urges to overeat didn't work, did they? Those diets you've been on may have given you temporary relief from overweight, but your appetite always came back and compelled you to overeat. That's when the weight returned.

Since the old-fashioned, unnatural approach to weight loss hasn't worked for you, why not give my method a try? After you use this natural system, you'll never want to use conventional diets again.

ào ào ào

THE *FATS* FEELINGS

S ome people's food cravings remain constant; for example, they always crave ice cream. Other people go through "food kicks," craving peanut butter one week, blue cheese dressing the next week, and chocolate bars the following week. Neither situation is an accident nor a coincidence. If your emotional issue remains unaddressed, your food craving will remain constant. If your emotional issues change, so will your food cravings. The only parallel between both the constant and the changing food cravings is this: there is some underlying emotional issue crying out for your attention.

By "emotional issue," I don't necessarily mean a deep psychological matter requiring therapy. Food cravings often stem from basic unmet needs for fun, excitement, or love—issues most would consider "normal" and within our power to self-heal.

Studies confirm what many of us know from personal experience: overweight and chronically dieting people use food to sedate troubling emotions. For example:

— One survey confirmed that overweight people report, more than thin or normal-weight people, that they eat when they're anxious or depressed. In fact, the more overweight the survey respondent was, the more likely he or she was to emotionally overeat.[1]

— Another study looked for past or present psychiatric diagnoses among 54 obese people enrolled in a weight-reduction program. Among these 54 subjects, the rates for depression and other mood disorders were five times greater than those found in the general population.[2]

— In a similar study, researchers compared responses to anxiety in obese and normal-weight people. The obese subjects frequently turned to food to counteract anxiety. In contrast, the normal-weight subjects shunned food while under duress.[3]

— Compulsive overeaters sometimes say their lives are more stressful than those of other people. One study partially supports this complaint. Researchers measured the number of stressful life events of adolescent compulsive overeaters, and compared this number with a sample of adolescents who didn't overeat. The overeaters had experienced 250 times more life-stress events than the normal-weight teenagers.[4]

— In a study of female college coeds, researchers noted that obese students ate more during final exams week, while normal-weight students ate less.[5]

This summary of studies is not intended to point an accusatory finger at overweight individuals. Instead, it's a confirmation for anyone who struggles with food cravings whenever she or he feels lonely, upset, or bored. If this situation applies to you, know that you're definitely not alone, and there *is* a way out, as you will discover as you read on.

Emotional issues connected to food cravings usually fall into one of these categories:

+ Stress, tension, anxiety, fear, or impatience
+ Depression or feeling blue
+ Feeling tired, having low energy levels
+ Unmet needs for fun, play, excitement, or recreation.
  Too much work and not enough play
+ A desire for love, affection, appreciation, romance,
  or sexual satisfaction
+ Anger, resentment, bitterness, or frustration
+ Emptiness, insecurity, or a desire for comfort

In my book, *Losing Your Pounds of Pain: Breaking the Link Between Abuse, Stress, and Overeating*, I discussed at length the four emotions underneath emotional overeating: Fear, Anger, Tension, and Shame (FATS).

The initial letter, *F,* signifies that Fear is the root emotion in the FATS feelings. Anger, Tension, and Shame are all extensions of Fear. We feel Anger because we fear losing love in the form of something or someone valuable to us; we feel Tension because we are afraid of trusting or because we've walked away from our Divine path; we feel Shame because we fear we are inadequate.

These FATS feelings are the primary triggers for emotional overeating. Overwhelming desires to eat stem from one of these four FATS feelings.

As a psychotherapist, I feel it's important to be honest with ourselves about our emotions. We need to face the emotion and then move on. I never recommend overanalyzing one's life, or viewing oneself as a victim. Yet, the source of so much needless emotional pain is the unwillingness to face an uncomfortable feeling. No one enjoys admitting, "Oh, yes, I feel insecure." But the alternative—not admitting it—is so much worse!

When we deny our strong emotions, they grow stronger. As they gain strength, they also seek outlets. Denied emotions manifest themselves in many unpleasant ways, including food cravings, physical aches or illnesses, depression, anxiety, phobias, and sleep disorders.

The bottom line is this: as unpleasant as it is to face a negative emotion, the alternative is even more so. Everyone gets angry, upset, or jealous at some time—there's no question about it. Sometimes life circumstances or our personal choices make it tough to stay centered in peace. In reality, the only legitimate issue is whether we choose to deal with these emotions now or later.

THE FOUR PRIMARY EMOTIONS
BEHIND EMOTIONAL OVEREATING

FEAR: Insecurity; walking on eggshells; generalized fears; abandonment fears; existential fears; control issues; sexual fears; worry; anxiety; depression; intimacy fears

ANGER: Toward another person; toward an injustice; toward self; feeling betrayed; feeling ripped-off; feeling abused

TENSION: Stress; frustration; old anger turned into bitterness or resentment; jealousy; impatience; overwork without an emotional release such as fun

SHAME: Self-blame; low self-esteem; self-loathing; lack of trust in one's own competence or goodness; assuming other people won't like you; feeling less than others; feeling like you don't deserve good

When we bottle up our strong emotions, it's akin to putting a cork on a vinegar-and-baking soda combination. The ignored emotion doesn't go away; it intensifies. The more we try to ignore a feeling, the stronger it grows! It's so much easier to face the music while the emotion is still in a "fixable" stage.

That's why I really have an appreciation for food-craving analysis. You start by identifying the food you crave and work backwards, like a detective. Once you've identified the particular food; say, "rocky road ice cream," the underlying emotion stares you plainly in the face: You are feeling frustrated or angry and feel you are missing out on something, and it's making you depressed.

The truth of that underlying emotion hits most of us between the eyes. We instantly recognize, "Yes, that is the emotional issue I've been struggling with." This recognition may inspire you to investigate further and take the healthy second step of asking yourself, "What makes me so frustrated or angry?" "What do I feel I'm missing out on?" and "Why am I taking my anger out on myself?" Usually, the answers appear right away.

Our denial system is incredibly effective in shielding us from honestly facing ourselves. Denial stems from a fear of admitting: "Yes, this bothers me." The consequences of such an admission can be even scarier, though, as in: "Now I must take responsibility for making changes to correct the situation." Change is frightening, because we fear our situation might worsen instead of improve.

Inertia and fears keep us from examining underlying issues that create food cravings. Since this denial keeps us from seeing these seemingly obvious issues, we often need to have them pointed out to us. It's relatively easy to recognize other people's issues; it's much tougher to be objective with ourselves. By learning to interpret your food cravings, you will be able to more readily discover these issues yourself.

Just honestly admitting to yourself, "Yes, this is the emotion underneath my food craving," is such a tremendous relief! It feels so good to come clean with yourself, doesn't it? That emotional relief then reduces, or even eliminates, the urge to overeat.

Physically Based Cravings

Sometimes, we'll crave a food because our body is screaming out for nutrients, such as B or C vitamins, or protein. Our body is depleted, so the craving is an example of the body's marvelous ability to ensure that its needs are met. These are physically based cravings.

Yet, on close examination, even these cravings are rooted in emotions. Tension, the third FATS feeling, is the physical manifestation of stress in our lives. Stress leads to lifestyle choices which, in turn, lead to nutritional deprivation. Three of my clients discovered how stress-filled lifestyles robbed their bodies of energy and nutrients, triggering food cravings:

— Dianna's hectic schedule convinced her that she had "no time to exercise." Without regular physical activity, Dianna always felt sluggish and tired. Instead of solving the problem with a brisk walk or a bike ride, Dianna would eat foods to feel "peppier."

— Marcia's high-pressure job contributed to her overall feeling of tension and inability to relax. Marcia craved and ate bags of potato chips and pretzels to gnaw away her anxiety and tension. Junk foods rob our bodies of B vitamins, because empty calories require nutrients for digestion. When you use nutrients for digestion, yet don't replace them, you become nutrient-deficient. Marcia was continually vitamin-deficient and therefore, continually hungry!

— Brenda used alcohol to calm her nerves. As you'll read in Chapters 8 and 16, excessive alcohol consumption contributes to lowered levels of the brain chemical, *serotonin*. When serotonin is low, the usual result is a craving for carbohydrates—which is exactly what Brenda struggled with. Her appetite for breads and pasta was out of control, and Brenda was most unhappy with her weight.

Yes, Dianna, Marcia, and Brenda all suffered from physically based food cravings. But the root of their nutrient deficiency was Tension, one of the FATS feelings.

Tension also increases the amount of brain chemicals that lead to overeating. Dr. Sarah Leibowitz of Rockefeller University found that the hormone, *cortisol,* stimulates production of a brain chemical called *neuropeptide Y.* This brain chemical is a chief factor in turning our carbohydrate cravings on and off. Here's the tension link: we produce more cortisol when we are tense! Even worse, Leibowitz also reports that neuropeptide Y also makes the body hang on to the new body fat we produce (apparently this is some ancient biological throwback to the cave days). In other words, tension not only triggers carbohydrate cravings, it also makes it more difficult to lose any ensuing weight.

What Do You Crave?

If you were at one of my workshops or in the audience when I was on a television or radio talk show, I could have interpreted your food craving for you. You'd just tell me the food you were craving—say, a cheeseburger with extra cheese, sauce, and dill pickles, and I'd tell you exactly what it meant. I'd ask you whether you preferred a hamburger bun that is soft or toasted and whether you craved extra salt and pepper on the patty. From your answers, I could tell you what this craving meant.

The information in this book, however, will allow you to conduct your own food-craving interpretations. I'll teach you the meaning behind each type of food, so you can analyze—and reduce—your own appetite. Each chapter discusses a different food group, and there is a food-craving chart in the last chapter of the book that references some of the most frequently craved foods.

But first, I want to continue exploring the appetite mechanism. Let's explore the differences between emotional and physical hunger, and some of the life situations that most often trigger emotional overeating.

EMOTIONAL HUNGER:
TRAITS, TRIGGERS, AND TRIUMPHS

"Help me! I'm hungry all the time and I can't stop eating!"

The woman in my office was crying from frustration over her out-of-control appetite. Ruth was a 37-year-old registered nurse with a wealth of knowledge about nutrition and biology. She couldn't understand, with all her physiological training and education, why her eating habits were so poor. As Ruth so succinctly put it, "It feels like my body and my appetite are betraying me. I keep promising myself that I'll eat better and lose weight, but my mouth and stomach seem to have other ideas!"

Ruth described how her appetite and eating seesawed. She'd read about a new diet and would strictly adhere to it. With each new diet, Ruth would always lose five or ten pounds. But then something would upset her, such as an unruly patient at the hospital where she worked, or her supervisor ordering her to work a double shift, or a problem in her marriage. At those times, Ruth's commitment to weight loss would dissipate, replaced by sudden and intense cravings for cookies, cake, and ice cream.

Ruth binged in secret, private places. That way, no one would see her, criticize her, or stop her rapid ingestion of high-fat sweets. Ruth ate in her car, in the bathroom, even in the laundry room. By the time she came to see me for help, Ruth's self-esteem was practically ripped to shreds from her shame and frustration.

"I know I'm smart," Ruth told me, "and I'm good at my nursing job. I help save people's lives every day." Then her cheeks flushed red. Ruth pounded her right fist on the easy chair arm and gritted her teeth. "So why—if I'm so damn smart—why can't I just quit overeating?!"

Caring for Everyone Else

Ruth was right. She *was* good at her job. Like many compulsive overeaters, Ruth was excellent at helping other people but terrible when it came to helping herself. I've worked with many helping professionals such as Ruth, who are paid to nurse, doctor, teach, give therapy, or just to serve other people. Helping professionals are attracted to their professions because they learned young how to meet other people's needs.

In Ruth's case, she was the oldest of three. Her mother was chronically ill, and her father spent most of his time at work or in his home office. Ruth's "job" was chief family caretaker. She gave her mother medicine and sponge baths. She helped her little sisters with their homework. Ruth even shopped and cooked the family meals, and delegated her siblings' chores. At age 12, Ruth lived the role of a "Mom."

In high school, Ruth continued her ultra-responsible persona, excelling in school and receiving straight A's." She went straight into nursing college, partly out of duty and partly to get away from her family. That's when Ruth first began to gain weight.

"I had never lived away from home before," she recalled. "I was so, so lonely, and the pressures of school were almost too much to handle. All that memorization, anatomy, and everything. It was horrible!" Ruth's memories of college are a blur of final exams, cheeseburgers, and pizzas. By the time she graduated, the young woman had gained 35 pounds.

The next 15 years saw Ruth become a registered nurse, get married, and have two children. She also tried diets, gyms, a hypnotist, home exercise equipment, and appetite-suppressant pills. Still, her weight and eating were out of control.

Out of Control, Out of Touch

I had a suspicion. To check it out, I asked Ruth to describe how her shoes felt on her feet. How the waistband of her pants felt. How her bra strap felt. When she would focus on her own bodily sensations, Ruth was surprised to find that her bra straps were digging into her shoulders and back, and that her bra underwire was poking into her skin. She expressed surprise when she noted that her waistband felt too tight, and her shoes seemed overly small and narrow.

But I wasn't surprised because I've seen it so many times before. Ruth was tuned out, unaware of her own bodily sensations. She'd focused all her attention on other people. That's why Ruth was an excellent nurse, mother, and caretaker. She put 100 percent of her energy into anticipating and fulfilling other people's needs! And because all her energy was outer-directed, Ruth was deaf, dumb, and blind toward her own needs.

She didn't notice her pinching shoes and bra straps any more than she noticed her appetite. Ruth was out of touch with the true physical sensations of hunger and fullness. She could eat and eat and eat and eat until she was as stuffed as a Thanksgiving turkey. But Ruth couldn't "feel" a sense of fullness since her awareness was directed outward.

Likewise, Ruth's signals of hunger were distorted. She would confuse emotional hunger, marked by stress and anger, with physical hunger.

For many clients such as Ruth, therapy has involved getting them back in touch with their own bodies. I asked Ruth to close her eyes, take a few deep breaths, and describe to me the feeling of her feet on the floor, her legs against the chair, her bottom resting on the chair, and her hands and fingers against the chair's velour upholstery. I asked her to tell me what her arms felt like, what her jaw felt like, and what her neck felt like.

I asked her to focus on herself for once, as a means of reacquainting Ruth with her own bodily sensation and as a way of learning to distinguish between emotional and physical hunger. Once someone learns the difference, the emotional hunger loses much of its power. The appetite becomes more normalized, giving that person more control, and lessening the chance of binge-eating.

THE 8 TRAITS OF EMOTIONAL HUNGER

Emotional and physical hunger can feel identical, unless you've learned to identify their distinguishing characteristics. The next time you feel voraciously hungry, look for these signals that your appetite may be based on emotions rather than true physical need. This awareness may head off an emotional overeating episode.

Emotional Hunger:

1. *Is sudden*. One minute you're not thinking about food, the next minute you're starving. Your hunger goes from 0–60 m.p.h. within a short period of time.

2. *Is for a specific food*. Your cravings are for one certain type of food, such as chocolate, pasta, or a cheeseburger. With emotional eating, you feel you *need* to eat that particular food. No substitute will do!

3. *Is "above the neck."* An emotionally based craving begins in the mouth and the mind. Your mouth wants to taste that pizza or chocolate doughnut. Your mind whirls with thoughts about your desired food.

Physical Hunger:

Is gradual. Your stomach rumbles. One hour later, it growls. Physical hunger gives you steadily progressive clues that it's time to eat.

Is open to different foods. With physical hunger, you may have food preferences, but they are flexible. You are open to alternative choices.

Is based in the stomach. Physical hunger is recognizable by stomach sensations. You feel a gnawing, a rumbling, emptiness, and even pain in your stomach with physical hunger.

4. *Is urgent.* Emotional hunger urges you to eat NOW! There is a desire to instantly ease emotional pain with food.

Is patient. Physical hunger would prefer that you ate soon, but doesn't command you to eat right at that instant.

5. *Is paired with an upsetting emotion.* Your boss yelled at you. Your child is in trouble at school. Your spouse is in a bad mood. Emotional hunger occurs in conjunction with an upsetting situation.

Occurs out of physical need. Physical hunger occurs because it has been four or five hours since your last meal. You may experience light-headedness or low energy if overly hungry.

6. *Involves automatic or absent-minded eating.* Emotional eating can feel as if someone else's hand is scooping up the ice cream and putting it into your mouth ("automatic eating"). You may not notice that you've just eaten a whole bag of cookies ("absent-minded eating").

Involves deliberate choices and awareness of the eating. With physical hunger, you are aware of the food on your fork, in your mouth, and in your stomach. You conciously choose whether to eat half your sandwich, or the whole thing.

7. *Does not cease, even when the body is full.* Emotional overeating stems from a desire to cover up painful feelings. You stuff yourself to deaden your troubled emotions, and you will eat second and third helpings, even though your stomach may hurt from over-fullness.

Stops when satisfied. Physical hunger stems from a desire to fuel and nourish the body. As soon as that intention is fulfilled, you stop eating.

8. *Promotes guilt about eating.* The paradox of emotional overeating is that you eat to feel better, and then end up berating yourself for eating cookies, cakes, or cheeseburgers. You promise to atone ("I'll exercise, diet, skip meals, and so on—tomorrow!")

Is based on eating as a necessity. When the intent behind eating is based in physical hunger, there's no guilt or shame. You realize that eating, just like breathing oxygen, is a requisite ingredient of life.

Breaking Free from Emotional Overeating

It takes practice and patience to consistently identify whether your hunger is emotional or physical. If you've experienced emotional hunger, you know how overwhelming that urge to eat can be. Even if you've sworn to yourself, "I'm not going to overeat," emotional hunger changes everything. Even the most committed health fanatic finds oneself drawn toward the refrigerator, desperately digging for something to fulfill overwhelming cravings.

Let's break the horrible hold that emotional hunger has over your appetite and eating habits! Let's give you back the freedom and control to say, "No, I refuse to overeat!" The way to do just that is to take these five steps the next time you feel hungry:

5 Steps to Reduce Emotional Hunger

The next time you find yourself feeling extremely hungry, these steps may help you:

1. *Impose a 15-minute cooling-off period.* Tell yourself you cannot eat for 15 minutes. After that time, if you still feel like eating, you'll be free to do so. But during that 15 minutes, you'll be completing the other four steps, and your appetite will likely be reduced to the point where you won't want to overeat.

2. *Get away from food.* Leave the house if you must, but definitely stay away from the kitchen during the next 15 minutes. Emotional overeating often leads to "automatic" and "absent-minded" eating, where you don't realize how much food you are eating. An eating binge may be avoided simply by getting away from food. Sometimes, I'd have to destroy the food I was craving. It wasn't enough to throw the box of cookies away, because I'd simply dig the box out of the trash can. Then I'd feel even more disgusted with myself. During those times, it's better to put the food in the garbage disposal (this costs less than psychotherapy or treating weight-related illnesses!) or pour it directly out of its container and into the trash can so that the food is rendered inedible.

3. *If you are having "mouth hunger," brush your teeth and drink a large glass of water (but still stay away from the kitchen for 15 minutes!).* By cleansing your mouth, you can get rid of the taste of chocolate, cheeseburgers, or cookies or whatever else you're craving, and help reduce your emotional appetite. The water will also help if you are confusing thirst with hunger (which occurs with surprising frequency).

4. *Ask yourself, "Am I feeling Fear, or its manifestations of Anger, Tension, or Shame?"* You don't need to go into deep intro-spection over this question. Usually, the answer pops in your mind instantly, like one of those "magic 8 balls" with answers floating in the window. You'll ask the question, and you'll hear the reply in your mind pretty quickly: "Yes, you're worried about your finances," "Yes, you feel insulted by your mother's words," or "Yes, you're jealous of the way he looked at that other woman."

Just the act of honestly admitting one's feelings is usually enough to relieve the urgency associated with emotional hunger. Emotional hunger reflects an imperative need to disguise or mask awareness of a painful truth, thought, or feeling. It's the equivalent of stick-ing your fingers in your ears when you don't want to hear some-thing! But if you've already admitted your true feelings to yourself, you won't feel the need to run for cover in the refrigerator.

5. *Replace the FATS feelings with self-love.* Metaphysical lecturer/author Marianne Williamson reminds us that we heal fear by pouring love on it. When you fill yourself with love, there is no room for negative emotions to exist. Re-member the times in your own life when you were blissfully enjoying the feelings of romantic love? Remember how, dur-ing those moments, you had no desire to overeat? Let's return to that feeling right now with these two powerful steps:

a. ***Look for a butterfly feeling in your stomach.*** Concentrate on your gut emotions, and search for any sign of a pleasant, light sensation. This fluttering is much like the happy feeling you get right before something wonderful is about to happen—the same sense that you'd get if your name was just announced as a contest winner, or the way you felt on a childhood holiday morning just prior to opening a gift.

It is the sense of love and fun that is always with us. Notice this feeling, and ask it to expand within you. Imagine yourself being swept high above all problems, riding on your butterfly feelings to a moment when all you feel is love, peace, and a sense of playful anticipation. Once you try this step, you'll know exactly what I mean.

b. ***Stay in love with this moment.*** Here is an affirmation that will fill you with peace of mind if you declare it over and over. It represents your new FATS feelings:

"I Forgive, Accept, and Trust my Self (FATS)."

The five steps listed above are simple and powerful. You will appreciate the immediacy with which they heal constant cravings. To me, the butterfly feelings expand into a sensation of deep romantic love, something more delicious than any chocolate I've ever eaten. With this feeling, I experience a peace that almost magically fixes whatever problems are around me. When I'm serene, I'm much more productive and creative, and people treat me with love and helpfulness. What a wonderful alternative to Fear, or its manifestations of Anger, Tension, or Shame!

I recommend photocopying the following abbreviated list of the five steps and carrying it in your wallet or purse.

THE FIVE STEPS TO REDUCE FATTENING FEELINGS

1. Decide not to eat for 15 minutes.
2. Get away from food, or destroy the food.
3. Brush your teeth or drink water to get rid of "mouth hunger."
4. Ask yourself: "Am I feeling Fear, or its manifestations of Anger, Tension, or Shame?"
5. Replace the FATS feelings with self-love by:
   a. looking for, and expanding, a butterfly feeling in your gut; and
   b. affirming over and over, "I Forgive, Accept, and Trust my Self."

© Doreen Virtue

Food Groups/Food Cravings

Our bodies, minds, and emotions are marvelously complex creations, and the appetite is no exception. As you'll read in the next three chapters, there are fascinating reasons why we experience emotional hunger. There are no accidents or coincidences concerning food cravings. If, as I've mentioned before, you get a sudden yearning for a particular food, there's a definite reason for that craving.

Here are the top ten food categories most commonly craved during emotional hunger. For some people, the food craving remains consistent throughout their life; for example, they always crave sweets. Other people go through phases. They crave cheeseburgers one month and the next month finds them on a Chinese food kick. Many women crave carbohydrates such as bread, salty potato chips, nuts, alcohol, and chocolate during their menstrual cycle. Some crave more carbohydrates in the winter. Each food category and eating style is addressed in separate chapters throughout this book.

THE 10 FOOD CATEGORIES MOST COMMONLY CRAVED

1. *Chocolate:* Brownies, cake, candy, cereal, cheesecake, cookies, doughnuts, frosting, frozen yogurt, fudge, ice cream, milkshakes, pudding, syrup, truffles.

2. *Dairy Products:* Blue cheese dressing, butter, buttermilk dressing, cheese, cream cheese, cottage cheese, dip, ice cream, mayonnaise, milk, pudding, sour cream, white sauces.

3. *Nuts and Crunchy Snack Foods:* Chips (all types), crackers, crispy fries, crispy noodles, nuts, crispy onion rings, croutons, crunchy bread sticks, ice cream cones, nuts, peanut butter (smooth or crunchy), popcorn, pretzels.

4. *Liquids:* Alcohol (beer, distilled spirits, wine); coffee; cola (diet and regular).

5. *High-Fat Foods:* Burgers, soft french fries.

6. *Spicy or Highly Seasoned Foods:* Ethnic foods: Indian food, Indonesian food, Italian food, Mexican food, Thai food. Pickled foods: dill, sweet, and bread-and-butter pickles; pickled herring; pickled eggs. Smoked foods, including fish and meat; spices and condiments: cinnamon, curry, dill, garlic, mint, mustard, onion, pepper, peppermint, salt, sugar, vinegar.

7. *Bread and Starch Products:* Bagels, biscuits, bread, cereal, crepes, granola, pancakes, pasta, potatoes—baked or mashed, rice, rolls, soft bread sticks, waffles.

8. *Cookies, Cakes, and Pies:* Includes doughnuts and pastries.

9. *Candy:* All non-chocolate candy, including butterscotch, caramel, coffee-flavored candy, fruit-flavored candy, gum drops, hard candies, jelly beans, licorice; mints, nougats, red-hots, toffee, vanilla.

10. *Fruits, Vegetables, and Salads:* Fresh fruits and vegetables, jams and jellies, juice, pies, purées, salads (including fruit salad), bean salad, vegetable salad, sauces (such as applesauce).

ã ã ã

WHAT TYPE OF
EMOTIONAL EATER ARE YOU?

B y this point, you've probably decided whether or not your food cravings and overeating are based on uncomfortable emotions. Let's look at your eating style a little closer.

Not all emotional eaters are alike. There are five distinct styles of emotional eating; perhaps one or more of these styles describes *you*. In addition, some people comprise a blend of two, three, or four styles. Many people tell me they possess characteristics from all five eating styles! Thirty-one different blends of emotional overeating are possible.

Why is this important to know? As I've said before, it's important to tailor your self-help regimen to fit your unique lifestyle, personality, and desires. Nothing else will do! The eating or weight-loss plan that fits your mother, sister, best friend, or co-worker may not fit you. They may be eating for entirely different reasons than you are. Your eating style is one of the most important factors to consider when adopting a successful nutritional program that you'll maintain for a lifetime.

You've undoubtedly read or heard that *consistency* is the most important aspect of healthy living—regularly eating a nutritionally balanced meal, exercising several times a week, and so on. But unless your eating regimen suits your personality, it will feel as unnatural as ill-fitting clothes or shoes, and you will eventually abandon anything that feels uncomfortable.

Here's a quiz that I devised many years ago to help those, like you, who wish to understand themselves better. I've given this quiz on TV and radio shows throughout the country many times, and audience members consistently report gaining great insights from it.

When answering each question, try not to judge yourself or in any way color your answers to fit what you think your ideal eating style ought to look like. I'm sure that you are very educated about what constitutes a healthful eating style—as we discussed in Chapter One, people who struggle with weight are usually self-taught nutritional experts.

You'll gain the most from this quiz by boldly answering each question with the first answer that pops into your mind.

QUIZ: WHAT'S YOUR EATING STYLE?

True or False:

1. I tend to overeat one or two certain types of food.

2. Once I have one bite of a food such as a certain type of dessert, dairy product, baked good, or salty junk food, my eating habits and appetite go out of control.

3. I sometimes worry—often without justification—that I won't get enough to eat.

4. I crave certain flavors or types of foods, and sometimes the only way to make the cravings go away is to eat whatever I have the desire for.

5. I have gone to extreme lengths (e.g., driven several miles out of my way; spent excessive money, etc.) to get the food I'm craving.

6. I only overeat when I'm feeling a strong emotion, such as anger or depression.

7. Right after work, I head straight for food.

8. I tend to eat whenever I'm bored.

9. Sometimes, out of the blue, I'll find that I am incredibly hungry.

10. I feel uncomfortable openly displaying or talking about my feelings.

11. I wish I were a more confident and strong person.

12. Just when I lose enough weight to start receiving compliments or admiring glances, I tend to start putting the weight back on again.

13. For the most part, I want to lose weight to please my spouse, parent, lover, or some other person.

14. I'm almost to the point where I've given up hope that I'll ever lose my excess weight; maybe I'm meant to be overweight.

15. My weight makes me feel bad about myself, and when I gain weight, I feel like a failure.

16. I never seem to have enough time to eat right or exercise.

17. I'm so busy that some days I wonder if I'll drop from exhaustion.

18. I seem to be working harder these days and getting less accomplished.

19. The only way I can unwind most of the time is when I'm eating.

20. Food is a great pick-me-up when I'm feeling drained but feel that I need to keep going.

21. My weight changes during the seasons; I'm one weight in the summer and a different weight during the winter.

22. Eating is one of the few pleasures left in my life.

23. Sometimes when I'm lonely, I'll nibble on whatever's handy.

24. Usually when I diet, I'll eventually stop caring whether I lose weight or not. That's when I return to overeating.

25. I often go back for second or third helpings of "diet," low-fat, or low-calorie foods.

Scoring:

Add up the "true" answers you gave for the preceding questions, and read the interpretations corresponding to your answers:

Note: There are no right or wrong answers to this quiz. It is designed to help you better understand your eating style. Understanding yourself is always an important step in making desired behavior changes. Many people find that they exhibit more than one Emotional Eating Style; some people exhibit all five styles. After scoring your quiz, read the information related to every emotional eating style relevant to you.

+ If you answered "True" to 3 or more of Questions 1 through 5, you are a "Binge Eater."

+ If you answered "True" to 3 or more of Questions 6 through 10, you are a "Mood Eater."

+ If you answered "True" to 3 or more of Questions 11 through 15, you are a "Self-Esteem Eater."

+ If you answered "True" to 3 or more of Questions 16 through 20, you are a "Stress Eater."

+ If you answered "True" to 3 or more of Questions 21 through 25, you are a "Snowball Effect Eater."

The Five Emotional Eating Styles

Did you find yourself falling into more than one eating style? Many people do. After all, we're multidimensional creatures that don't fit into a single pigeonhole. We are complex blends of our past experiences, present situations, heredity, emotions, thoughts, beliefs, and behaviors. We evolve and change, usually driven by desires to improve ourselves, and sometimes thwarted by life's roadblocks. All these factors influence our eating styles, and what holds true for you today may be entirely different one year from now.

Although there are 31 different possibilities (made up of various blends of the five main styles) of the categories described below, they are still too simplistic to fully capture the intricacies of emotional overeating. Yet, these 31 eating styles are about 30 more descriptions than in most diet books I've picked up.

In the typical diet book, we get pat answers and one-size-fits-all prescriptions. I used to feel perplexed by diet doctors' advice, such as, "If you're feeling upset, stay out of the kitchen." No other mention of, or suggestions about, emotional overeating exists in most of these books!

When my book, *The Yo-Yo Syndrome Diet: Why Your Weight Goes Up and Down, and How to Keep It Down for Good,* was first published in 1989, it was considered radical! Three-fourths of the book was devoted to the subject of emotional overeating, and traditional diet advice only comprised a minor part of the book. Today, it's accepted as common knowledge that emotions play a role in overeating and unhealthful eating.

With that information in mind, here are the five core emotional eating styles:

1. *The Binge Eater*—This is a very black-and-white eating style—you either are a Binge Eater or you're not. Those who are Binge Eaters will instantly recognize this description. Those who aren't Binge Eaters will think this is an outlandish description.

   Certain foods trigger overeating in Binge Eaters. Those foods are often referred to as "binge foods." Binge foods commonly are made from refined white flour or sugar—foods such as sweets, pastas, and breads. Different theories have tried to explain the binge-food phenomenon. Some experts believe

Binge Eaters become anxious as a result of blood sugar fluctuations triggered by eating high-glucose foods. This anxiety leads to a cycle of binge-eating to relieve the condition.

Many Binge Eaters find that the only way to keep their appetite under control is by avoiding their binge food altogether. This is also a useful therapeutic approach, because often the binge food keeps a lid on the person's underlying emotional issues. When the binge food is removed from their availability, the emotions are free to come forward for resolution. Binge Eaters benefit from interpreting their cravings for the binge food, using the methods in this book.

2. *The Mood Eater*—This is a person who overeats in response to strong emotions. Often, the Mood Eater is an exquisitely sensitive individual who is very compassionate and empathetic with respect to other people. Mood Eaters are sensitive to other people's feelings and intuitively know when something is troubling another person. Often, the Mood Eater is employed in a helping profession, such as teaching, counseling, or medicine.

Mood Eaters are so engulfed by the emotions that they've absorbed from other people that their own feelings are sublimated or ignored. They may also feel overwhelmed by the prospect of adding their own strong emotions onto their already-full plate. So they eat in order to manage their emotional capacity.

Although Mood Eaters are highly capable caretakers of others, they sometimes neglect themselves altogether. Sometimes, this realization upsets Mood Eaters, as they realize that they are doing all the work, and no one is attending to their needs. At those times, The Mood Eater feels unappreciated and resentful. They take out their frustration in the best way they know how—by eating.

Mood Eaters benefit by the methods outlined in the chapter on Extroverts (Chapter 7). Since Mood Eaters are externally oriented—focusing more on other people than on themselves—they can tune into their own feelings and become more inner-directed by interpreting their food cravings as they arise.

3. *The Self-Esteem Eater*—This is someone who uses food as a friend, a companion, and for entertainment. The Self-Esteem Eater has difficulties in interpersonal relationships. Often, Self-Esteem Eaters relate better to food, books, animals, and movies than they do to other people. They feel misunderstood and have been hurt by people who rejected or abandoned them. Many Self-Esteem Eaters are survivors of emotional, physical, or sexual abuse, and they learned in early childhood to distrust others.

Much of the Self-Esteem Eaters' struggle with food and weight stems from three issues:

— **They can't bear the thought of losing their closest friend: food.** The thought of giving up the overeating of ice cream, cookies, or cheeseburgers makes them feel cold and vulnerable. If they aren't able to use food for comfort, companionship, and solace, who or what can they turn to?

— **They have little confidence in their ability to lead a healthful lifestyle.** The Self-Esteem Eater is usually well read and informed about the importance of healthful eating and exercise. Their library may be stocked with health books. Yet they don't believe that they have the stamina or patience to consistently exercise. So they don't even try.

— **They beat themselves up by going on eating binges.** Self-Esteem Eaters struggle with the fourth FATS feeling: Shame. They question their self-worth, and deep down they wonder if something is wrong with them. During these times, they punish themselves by eating to the point where their stomach hurts. Self-Esteem Eaters don't believe that they deserve the benefits of having a fit and healthy body.

Self-Esteem Eaters benefit more from appropriate psychotherapy than from any particular style of eating. This is not to imply that something is wrong with Self-Esteem Eaters; rather, they just have the most to gain from this type of treatment.

Therapy will most likely be the first experience they have being emotionally vulnerable in front of another human being—that is, a skilled therapist. But when Self-Esteem Eaters find that the therapist doesn't reject them for being who they are, they will be able to connect with other people in their life. They can then develop friendships with people, and stop relying on food for companionship and comfort.

Self-Esteem Eaters also benefit from food-craving interpretation as a way of becoming more honest with themselves. When they face the truth behind the meaning of their food cravings, it's a first step toward easing the loneliness that haunts them. Self-honesty always increases one's self-esteem, and food-craving interpretation is a productive way of honestly coming to terms with parts of ourselves we may be afraid of facing.

4. *The Stress Eater*—This person overeats in response to the third FATS feeling: Tension. I've found that two life areas trigger Stress Eating: unhappiness with one's work life, and dissatisfaction with one's love life. Both life areas are difficult to change, and usually take time and effort to correct. Because we can't just snap our fingers and "fix" the love or work life, we overeat to ease the tension.

Stress Eaters usually have a wide range of food cravings, all intuitively chosen to ease their tension and frustration. They crave alcohol to manage their ever-taut nerves, coffee and cola to pump up their enthusiasm and energy, chocolate to ease their love-life disappointments, breads and dairy products to calm themselves down, and crunchy snack foods to control their anger.

Food-craving interpretation is one way of accessing the underlying sources of frustration so that they may be dealt with head-on. I also encourage Stress Eaters to add four essential ingredients to their life, which help with tension much more effectively than do foods or beverages:

a. ***Exercise.*** Please don't assume that I'm asking you to add one more responsibility to your already-full plate of things to do. I realize that it's a hassle to exercise. Still, exercise is one of the easiest ways to feel better, reduce stress, get more energy, control anger, and reduce the appetite. The best motivational tool I've ever found with respect to exercise is to develop a focused mindset that "exercise is a non-optional activity." Put exercise into the same category as your daily shower, and see it as something that you simply need to do. No ifs, ands, or buts!

b. ***Fun and Recreation.*** The number-one source of resentment is the feeling that everybody else gets to relax and have fun, while we're left with all the chores and responsibility. It's a powerful residual emotion left over from childhood. Many people feel that fun is a waste of time or a sign of weakness. Yet, fun—like exercise—is a necessity, not a luxury.

Would you like to feel as if you have two extra hours in the day? You'll get that feeling when you incorporate small daily doses of fun into your life. Fun recharges the soul and the spirit, giving you the energy and enthusiasm necessary to meet your responsibilities. Fun doesn't have to cost anything or take more than 10 or 15 minutes. The important thing is for you to give yourself permission to relax and enjoy yourself every day.

c. *Time Outdoors.* Stress Eaters usually lead whirlwind lifestyles. They're running at a dead heat from the moment they wake up until the time they go to bed at night. This harried pace leaves little time for noticing the simple and beautiful things in everyday life.

Here's an instant stress-buster, kind of a game you can play with yourself on a daily basis: When you are driving home from work or during your lunch hour, notice three things in nature. This could be a cloud, the sound of a bird singing, the reflection on a puddle of water, or the colors in a sunset.

If you really want to ease your tension, take a walk during your lunch hour or eat lunch outside (near grass or trees). Being in close proximity to nature is instantly stress-reducing. It calms our nerves, soothes our soul, and definitely slows us down. I suppose that's where the phrase, "Stop and smell the roses" came from.

d. *Spirituality.* When your heart feels full of love and gratitude, very few things can get on your nerves. People who are spiritual or religious are usually less vulnerable to earthly stressors, because they believe that everything will turn out for the best. Instead of sweating out the picayune details of everyday life, they "let go" and trust. This doesn't mean that they blindly accept the dictates of others. Spiritually guided persons are among some of the world's most successful individuals.

All four stress-reducing elements—exercise, having fun, spending time outdoors, and spirituality—can be combined effectively. For example, any type of outdoor activity, blended with meditation or prayer, will create an incredible boost of positive feelings and energy. And when you feel great, you won't crave food as much.

5. *The Snowball Effect Eater*—Think of a snowball rolling down a mountain, gaining momentum and size, and you'll have an idea of the Snowball Effect Eater's style. This person's determination to stick with a healthful eating and exercise program vacillates tremendously. Brenda's story typifies the struggle of a Snowball Effect Eater.

> Last December, Brenda was horrified when she saw a Polaroid picture of herself next to the Christmas tree. "Oh my gosh! Look how fat I look!" she exclaimed, and immediately made a New Year's resolution to lose weight.
>
> Her motivation to eat light was high after the holidays, so Brenda's dinner meals consisted of skinless chicken breasts, salads with fat-free dressing, and steamed rice. She lost six pounds in just a few weeks. Then, in mid-January, her husband decided to throw a Super Bowl party. Brenda volunteered to plan the snack menu. While preparing the pizza, chip dips, and other munchies, Brenda felt obligated as hostess to taste-test all the foods.
>
> After the Super Bowl, Brenda's incentive to diet decreased. She'd tasted those high-fat foods, and her mouth ached for more. So, her skinless chicken breast meal was now a fried half-of-a-chicken, complete with skin. Her fat-free salad now consisted of a small serving of lettuce, topped with huge portions of shredded cheese, bacon bits, croutons, and blue cheese dressing. She replaced the steamed rice with a huge baked potato, complete with butter and sour cream.

In Brenda's mind, she was still eating the basic "diet dinner menu" of chicken, salad, and a complex carbohydrate. She quit caring whether or not she lost weight, and barely noticed when she regained the six pounds.

Snowball Effect Eaters usually exhibit inconsistent motivation levels because their weight-loss efforts are externally motivated. Like Brenda, they declare themselves to be on a diet in response to some outer stimulus, such as a photograph, a spouse's comment, or too-tight jeans. However, these external sources of motivation just can't provide the steady stream of inspiration necessary for permanent changes in eating behavior. Internal motivation is necessary, with a focus on:

+ how much energy we have when we eat healthful foods,
+ how great it feels to have toned muscles,
+ how exercise eases our tension and worries,
+ how treating our bodies with respect leads to higher self-regard, and
+ the fact that the only opinion that matters, as far as our weight is concerned, is our own.

Brenda's black-and-white approach to weight loss also set her up for fluctuations both in her weight and in her motivation. Instead of saying, "Either I eat like a pauper, or I eat like a pig," Brenda could take a more conservative approach. Yes, it takes more time to lose weight using a moderate rather than a radical diet, but in the long run, we won't get those sharp swings in weight. So, instead of forcing ourselves to eat a bland, fat-free diet, it's more realistic to find a flavorful, low-fat menu that satisfies the taste buds as well as our nutritional requirements.

Snowball Effect Eaters benefit from food-craving interpretation because it keeps them focused on internal motivations for eating. Instead of viewing their food cravings as a sign of, "What's the use? I'm hungry, so I'll just abandon this stupid diet," they are more able to understand the underlying emotional significance of their cravings.

All five styles of emotional eating can employ food-craving interpretation as a means of reducing or eliminating intrusive desires to overeat. The more you understand about yourself, the more you're able to work with—instead of against—yourself. There's no need to fight yourself; that's an unloving thing to do that will only create depression and internal resistance. Instead, move toward gently understanding and accepting yourself.

As I wrote in *Losing Your Pounds of Pain: Breaking the Link Between Abuse, Stress, and Overeating*, trying to sublimate an emotion is like trying to ignore a child who desperately wants your attention. The child just screams louder and more urgently until the adult finally acknowledges him or her. Your emotions are just like that child. If you nurture and pay attention to them, they won't need to scream at you in the form of an overly active appetite.

So, really listen to your food cravings—they are part of your inner voice, and provide valuable information!

૱ ૱ ૱

APPETITE: THE DRIVE TO SURVIVE

T he appetite is an amazingly complex and yet, highly predictable phenomenon. I've always been interested in the
reasons why our appetites go wildly out of control. Most of
us are well fed, yet half the time we behave as if we were starving.

In university medical libraries, I uncovered some dusty old scientific journals where I found fascinating research about human and
animal appetite behavior. After poring through these studies, I was
awestruck by the amazing appetite we have been given. Scientists
call appetite, the inborn ability to self-regulate, "Nutritional Intelligence." I've summarized the highlights of this research for you
in this chapter. As you'll read, the appetite is a perfectly equipped
survival mechanism. Each of us, deep down, is an intuitively
knowledgeable nutritionist.

Infant Appetite Studies

Infants have an innate ability to regulate their caloric intake. No
one needs to teach a newborn how to diet—they naturally know
what their bodies need nutritionally. An interesting study of 37 newborns underscores this point. Researchers delivered premeasured
formula bottles containing milk that was either diluted or normal
to the babies' mothers, not telling them what type of formula the
babies were being fed. Researchers encouraged the mothers to
allow the babies to decide how much milk to consume.

The babies given diluted milk drank more, apparently to adjust their caloric and fat intake. Remarkably, both groups of babies ingested roughly the same number of calories and fat grams.[1]

Another infant study added further credence to the innate nutritional intelligence in humans. Researchers found a group of malnourished Jamaican children and gave them unlimited access to food. As you might expect, the children went on an eating binge! They indulged in 200 to 300 percent more food than a properly nourished child of the same age.

But, as soon as the Jamaican children's weight reached normal levels, their food intake dropped to the same rate as any well-fed American kid. The downward adjustment in the Jamaican children's caloric intake always occurred within 48 hours of their attaining a normal body weight. Thereafter, the children's weight stayed at a healthy and stable rate of growth. They didn't overcompensate and become obese little children, nor did they revert back to a starvation pattern. Given the option of unlimited feeding, these children self-regulated their weight at moderate levels.[2]

This self-regulation of calories is also evident in adults. In one well-controlled study, laboratory-bound subjects could eat as much as they wanted, but all food was prepared and delivered by the researchers. In that way, the researchers could measure all food intake.

Sometimes, unbeknownst to the subjects, they would receive low-calorie food, prompting an increase in food consumption. Whether they received high-calorie or low-calorie meals, the subjects' caloric intake always remained consistent. These results suggest some innate intelligence that guides us to eat enough to meet our caloric needs.[3]

Many of us have had this experience: you eat a low-cal frozen dinner and you're still hungry. So you eat another one. Now, the dinner has jumped from a light 300-calorie meal, to a 600-calorie meal. We could have, instead, enjoyed a "normal" meal and probably saved 100 calories to boot!

Feeding a Hungry Heart

The earliest stages of emotional eating are also evident during infancy. One study examined the intentions and motivations behind a mother's act of giving her baby a bottle. The mothers' reasons often had nothing to do with the baby's perceived hunger, but were, instead, a way of pacifying the child's fussiness.[4] Infants are soothed by a bottle, and both infant and child associate the bottle with emotional comfort. Perhaps milk's mood-altering properties (see Chapter 13) play a role in the bottle's calming effect. Regardless, the result is the same: the infant learns to pair food with love.

Researcher L.L. Birch has performed a number of studies that validate what most of us know to be true: when adults use food as a reward ("Here's some chocolate, Suzy. You've been such a good girl today, so you deserve a treat"), children learn to associate sweets with positive feelings. One study revealed that the mere act of an adult acting friendly while serving food to a child is enough to increase the child's preference for that food.[5]

The emotional link between love and food is also apparent in our vocabulary. Terms of endearment include "Sweetie Pie," "Honey Bun," "Pumpkin," "Sweetheart," "Lamb Chop," and "Muffin." You can probably think of some other delicious examples of pet names.

Valentine's Day and other emotion-filled holidays are also centered around food. Our birthdays are highlighted by cake and ice cream. Basically, we grow up associating celebrating with eating.

An interesting phenomenon revolves around falling in romantic love. When this happens, we often lose our appetite. We are so filled with bliss that we have no thoughts of eating. To me, this is the strongest evidence of the food/emotion link. If we can stay "in love" with our life, we will naturally find that we are unconcerned with food. And the way to fall in love with your life is by following your gut instincts, which will put you on the path to realizing all your dreams.

The Effect of Dieting on Appetite

Do diets trigger food cravings? Many researchers argue that the "good food/bad food" mentality creates an internal stress that does, in fact, inspire overeating.

Researcher Jean Harvey examined this question, both through a review of the literature about diet-craving connections and her own experimentation. She discovered no evidence that dieting increases our appetite.

In her review of the literature, Jean Harvey found no correlations between dietary restraint and cravings. Other studies reviewed by Harvey revealed no solid evidence that dieting increased the appetite beyond "normal" levels.

However, Harvey knew that current cultural wisdom is that "dieting leads to feelings of deprivation, which lead to food cravings." Eating-disorder therapists and researchers frequently cite anecdotal accounts of women who binge-eat in response to feelings of dieting deprivation. So, Harvey decided to test this theory scientifically, something that few of the eating-disorder theorists had done. She compared a group of subjects, one group on a very low-calorie diet, and one on a moderately low-calorie diet, over a period of 20 weeks. The very low-calorie diet group had no access to carbohydrates or high-fat foods.

She hypothesized that this very low-calorie group would have the greatest cravings, especially for carbohydrates or high-fat foods. Yet, both groups experienced decreases in cravings! The researcher concluded, "The main finding of this study was that participants on either a low-calorie diet or a very low-calorie diet program reported significant decreases in cravings for all types of foods."

Judith Rodin, a renowned eating-disorder researcher at Yale University, agreed with Jean Harvey. Rodin reported finding no significant correlations between dietary restraints and food cravings. This finding seemed to surprise Rodin, since she wrote, "We have speculated that women often have ambivalent feelings about foods seen as 'bad' or fattening, which may lead to experiencing them as more desirable." Other studies have yielded similar results: even though logic would tell us that diets make us hungrier, the empirical evidence doesn't back it up. The only types of diets associated with increased food cravings are those that restrict our caloric and fat intake below the level needed for basic survival.[6]

These studies make sense when you realize that food cravings are products of emotions, period. If our emotional issues are resolved, then our food cravings will change or dissipate. The only relationship between food cravings and dieting depends on whether your healthful eating and exercise habits increase your self-esteem. When you take good care of your body, you feel more energetic and proud. This positive result reduces the desire to overeat.

The only evidence I've found that would support the notion that dieting leads to overeating is the black-and-white thinking style of some dieters. They may eat one cookie and say to themselves, "I've blown my diet, so I may as well eat anything I want now!" Yet this type of overeating is again rooted in psychological, not physical, issues.

Dieting doesn't cause overeating. Unresolved emotions *do*!

Social Influences on Appetite

Do you eat more food than normal at crowded gatherings or at large dinner parties? Many people do, and studies show that the mere presence of other people stimulates overeating. In two studies, both male and female subjects ate significantly more food in group settings than when they were alone.[7]

Some of our food preferences are taught. One significant animal study closely examined how food tastes are acquired. Researchers taught rats, through aversive conditioning, using low levels of food poisoning, to hate one type of food and love another food type (yes, I know, I too wish researchers wouldn't do such things!). When these rats gave birth, the parent rats taught their babies to prefer the types of foods they had been conditioned to like.[8] Other animal species, including cats, monkeys, and chickens, teach their young about preferred food sources, as well.[9]

Of course, we humans are no exception, and our parents most likely taught us to enjoy many of the foods we eat today. Sometimes, these lessons came in the form of rewards or bribes. Think back and recall some of the lessons you learned about food as you were growing up. Ask yourself:

+ What eating habits did I learn by watching my family?
+ What types of food rewards did I receive, growing up?
+ Did I learn to associate food with good behavior?
+ Was food a part of our celebrations?
+ Do I crave any foods that were my favorite foods in childhood?
+ Who else in my family loved these foods? Could I have learned these cravings from that person?
+ Did I cook or bake with my mother? How did that close contact with my mother and food influence my feelings about cooking and eating today?
+ Did I learn any habits at the dinner table that influence my eating style today?
+ Did I ever compete with my siblings or other relatives to get my fair share of dinner or dessert?
+ If so, did that competition make me anxious about not getting enough to eat?

Reviewing the ways in which we developed our food preferences helps us understand why our eating habits sometimes defy logic. It also helps explain why it's so difficult to stick to an eating plan that doesn't suit our personality and lifestyle.

Environmental Influences on Appetite

Do you gain weight in the winter? Many of us do. The average American gains seven pounds between Thanksgiving and New Year's Day. You are probably already aware that the availability of high-fat foods and treats is part of the reason. Holiday stress, leading to overeating and under-exercising, is another culprit. Plus, if you live in a cold climate, winter clothing hides everything, which decreases the incentive to watch our figures!

Two other factors contributing to wintertime weight gain:

1. *Cold temperatures increase eating.* Studies on animals and humans confirm that when the temperature outside, or even within, the home, drops, occupants eat more frequently. The size of the meals doesn't increase; just the frequency with which we eat. So, instead of eating three square meals a day, we'll have several snacks and perhaps four meals.[10]

   Not only will we eat more during the winter, but studies show that we'll also work harder to be rewarded with food. In addition, we're more apt to settle for our least favorite foods when the mercury drops.[11] Cold temperatures seem to speed the rate of food digestion. This behavior quirk may also be a throwback to the days when we needed to fatten up for a long, harsh winter.

2. *Winter's decreased sunlight affects our appetite.* The primary brain chemical regulating carbohydrate (breads, starches, sweets, chocolates) cravings is highly sensitive to the amount of sunshine we take in. During the winter, when we're exposed to less sunlight, this important neurotransmitter, serotonin, is depleted. The body attempts to increase production of serotonin by sending signals to eat more carbohydrates. In Chapter 8, we'll talk about this *Seasonal Affective Disorder* syndrome in more depth.

Media Influences on Appetite

We've all seen them—the television and magazine advertisement photos of food so deliciously real you can practically smell and taste it. I remember one series of doughnut shop television commercials a few years ago. Against a black backdrop, pictures of chocolate-dripping doughnuts faded in and out. The voiceover actor sensually murmured, "Umm" and "Ahh" to the beat of the flashing images of frosting and candy sprinkles. Then the sounds of a conversation between a man and a woman were heard, simulating a couple watching the commercial and being so overcome by their cravings that they had to leave the house RIGHT AT THAT MOMENT to get one of those doughnuts. The ad showed no mercy!

Similar marketing ploys are used in pizza commercials featuring gooey, mouth-watering shots of mozzarella cheese, in ice cream ads that play up sensual licking scenes, in fast-paced ("This is the most fun!") soft-drink ads, and coffee-equals-love commercials. We consumers are bombarded with images that make us believe that food can change our moods for the better, lift our energy levels, elevate our social standing, and improve our love lives. Food is marketed as a cure-all for whatever ails us, and these commercials are the snake-oil salesmen of modern-day life!

Studies show that television viewing is linked to obesity, partly because the television viewer is inactive. I reported in *TV Guide* how people who watch television one to two hours a day are 150 percent more likely to be overweight than non-watchers. Those watching television more than three hours a day are 200 percent more likely to be overweight than non-viewers.

Inactivity only partially explains this TV-obesity link, though. Much of the problem, in my opinion, stems from viewing a steady stream of television characters eating food. Many of the dramas and sitcoms I see feature characters working out their life problems while sitting at a table eating dinner, ice cream, or some sort of snack food—behavior we may unwittingly model. Children who watch television snack-food commercials report greater preferences for those snacks than children who haven't seen such ads. [12]

Armed with this data showing links between eating and television viewing, some well-intentioned researchers have tried to influence children's eating preferences by showing them commercials about proper nutrition. Unfortunately, these ads had no impact—neither positive nor negative—on the children's food preferences. The researchers decided that their low-budget nutrition commercial couldn't complete with the slick, expensive advertisements of the snack-food industry.[13] Maybe if they'd presented an MTV-style "Vegetables-Are-Cool" campaign...

As a Baby Boomer, I grew up watching cartoonlike television commercials about those chocolate milk drinks, Ovaltine and Bosco. Could those ads have influenced the chocolate cravings I later struggled with?

As you think about your current food cravings, you might ask yourself:

+ What food advertisements do I recall from childhood?
+ Do any of those ads relate to the food cravings I have today?
+ What food advertisements am I exposed to today?
+ Is it possible that those advertisements influence my shopping or eating behavior?
+ Are there ways to reduce my exposure to food advertisements?
+ Do I need to monitor my children's exposure to food advertisements?
+ Would it be helpful to discuss these commercials with my children?

Self-Taught Cravings

We crave a certain food for one reason: to improve our mood or lift our level of energy. We desire that particular food in the hope that, after we eat it, we will experience peace of mind.

Usually, we've learned to associate that food with the feeling we're desiring. So in reality, we're not craving a food, we are instead craving a feeling. Studies show that the more times we are exposed to a food, the more we develop a preference for it—especially if that food has produced a positive feeling within us.

Although we appear to be born with innate desires for sweets, salt, and fat, we cannot possibly know how all foods taste. That is, until we try them, we don't know whether we'll enjoy or loathe foods as diverse as avocados, shrimp, or Mexican salsa. If we sample these foods, and experience positive feelings, such as happiness, contentment, a pleasant fullness, or an increase in our energy level, naturally we will want to eat that food again.

However, our food preferences are influenced by factors outside ourselves, as we've already seen in this chapter. We easily associate food with whatever circumstances occur while we're eating it. Our mother's mood and behavior, food commercials, and other people's food preferences have a profound unconscious effect on our appetite.

Many of our food cravings are actually rooted in childhood experiences. If you grew up receiving M & M's or chocolate cake as a reward for being "good," as an adult you'll likely treat yourself to these snacks when you want to celebrate, or console yourself. Similarly, if you were served one-too-many greasy pizzas while you were a lonely college student living away from home, you will probably be tempted to call for pizza delivery as an adult.

As children, we are especially vulnerable to family, social, and media influences when it comes to our eating behavior. But as adults, we're still exposed to external circumstances that can alter our food cravings. For example, if you have a horrible argument with your mate while eating prime rib at the neighborhood steak house, you'll probably hesitate before returning to that locale.

Premenstrual Cravings

"I never have problems with overeating, except once a month. Right before my period, I can't stay away from chocolate. It's so frustrating!" 33-year-old Wanda told me.

As is the case with Wanda, many women experience overwhelming food cravings that occur once a month like clockwork. These cravings are more physical than psychological, although the cravings certainly can trigger a lot of emotional distress. And that self-anger reflected in, "Why did I blow my diet!" can provoke an all-out eating binge.

There are three principal factors that account for premenstrual syndrome (PMS) cravings:

1. *Lowered serotonin levels.* Carbohydrate cravings for foods such as bread, pasta, chips, and sweets stem from the lowered levels of the brain chemical, serotonin, in women right before and during their menses. Those who suffer from intense PMS symptoms report the most acute problems dealing with food cravings, which can be attributed to the same source: low serotonin.[14]

2. *We burn more calories.* In addition, the metabolism increases during the premenstrual phase, and we actually burn calories a little faster. However, our increased appetite compensates for this, resulting in the fact that a premenstrual woman usually consumes more calories than she burns. This overeating tendency could also be nature's way of fattening us up, just in case we become pregnant.

3. *The smell of food is more intense.* We have a keener sense of smell right before our period, since all of our mucus—from the nose to the cervix—becomes thinner. Suddenly, the smells from the local bakery are overwhelmingly irresistible!

Pregnancy Cravings

I don't know where the rumors about pickles and ice cream originated, but I've met very few women who craved this rather unappealing combination of foods during pregnancy. During my first pregnancy, I had a different twist on the pickle-and-ice cream craving phenomenon. I have two children (actually, they're not children anymore, they're young men), and I was very young during my first pregnancy, with a job at the neighborhood deli. One of my duties was making prepared submarine sandwiches.

Every night, we employees were encouraged to help ourselves to any sandwiches that hadn't sold, and we were permitted to take home as many as we wanted. Help! What a terrible situation! This was the worst place a naive young pregnant woman could have ever worked. I would always rationalize that I was bringing the sandwiches home to my husband. But what I was really doing was hoarding food for myself like a pregnant squirrel storing nuts for the winter.

Our freezer was so full of sandwiches. And so was my stomach! I knew I was eating those sandwiches partly because I was so stressed from my job. For a little minimum-wage job, there was intense pressure to perform.

But mostly I was binge-eating sandwiches because I craved dill pickles. My typical sandwich was basically bread, wall-to-wall dill pickle slices, mustard, and a little meat and cheese. They were pickle sandwiches! But even though I craved—oh, heck, let's be honest—*I lived for* pickles, never once did it occur to me to mix them with ice cream.

For all the real-life and apocryphal experiences most of us have had with pregnancy cravings, there's not a whole lot of research on the topic. Most of the pregnancy research focus has been on calorie consumption, fetal nutritional requirements, and the ideal amount of weight gain prescribed for the expectant mom.

So I did research on my own, collecting the facts and data that are known about pregnancy and the psychoactive influences of food. We know, for example, that during the first trimester of pregnancy, the digestive tract transforms, and increased peptides (compounds containing amino acids) are secreted. These changes lead to "morning sickness," aversions to high-fat foods, and perhaps most importantly, fatigue.[15]

The sleepiness and low-energy levels during pregnancy are frustrating! Here you are, trying to rearrange your life to accommodate a brand-new baby. You have so many things to do to prepare the nursery, and you're bone-tired every day. So, in conducting my cravings research, I was pleasantly startled to discover this:

Pickles are stimulants!

It makes perfect sense, doesn't it? Of course a pregnant woman would crave a food that would stimulate her energy level. One study showed that pregnant women develop aversions to stimulants such as coffee and caffeinated soda, and develop cravings for milk, which is a sedative.[16] So, these tired mothers-to-be turn to pickles for energy.

Here's how it works: fermented foods and yeasts contain large amounts of tyramine, a natural food property that acts as a stimulant by raising blood pressure and increasing production of noradrenaline (a stimulant) in the brain. Other foods high in tyramine include cheese, pickled foods, tuna fish, sausages, wine, beer, soy sauce, sauerkraut, bananas, avocados, and liver.[17]

Hmm...come to think of it, I did eat sauerkraut and sausage when I was pregnant. But yuck; never liver!

Aversive Conditioning: From Craving to Loathing

Maybe, like me, you had this experience: you were a kid with the flu, a bad flu, complete with a stomachache, dizziness, nausea — the whole works. Then, your mom fixed you dinner. But because you were so sick, that dinner didn't much agree with you. Maybe the mere smell of cooking food was enough to nauseate you. Or maybe, like me, you ate Mom's dinner and then became completely nauseated.

Afterwards, you could never again smell, see, or taste that particular food without feeling ill. For me, it was salmon. Yep, my mom had made a beautiful salmon dinner, but because I ate it during one of my more memorable childhood sicknesses, I never wanted to see that pink-colored fish again.

It wasn't until I was in my late 20s that I had the courage to once again try some salmon. I expected to become instantly ill, as I had when I was 7 or 8 years old. Boy, was I shocked to find out that I loved the taste of salmon! It didn't nauseate me; it brought me pleasure! Today, salmon is one of my favorite foods.

Psychologists call this type of experience "one-trial learning." Normally, it takes humans and animals several experiences or "trials" before they pair an emotion with a neutral stimulus. Pavlov's dog, for example, had to hear the bell ring many times before he associated its sound with mealtime. Rats have to receive food in response to pressing a lever over and over before they learn that, if they want to eat, they must first press that lever.

In fact, it appears that pairing food aversions with illnesses is the quickest conditioning response there is. Whereas all other conditioning experiences take time for learning to occur, all organisms learn to dislike a food following an illness response *the first time it happens*!

Other remarkable studies show that rats learn to associate food with illness vicariously or, by example. In one study, rats ate a certain food and were immediately exposed to another rat who was very ill. Even though the just-fed rats were perfectly healthy, they associated that food with illness and refused to eat it in the future.[18]

Researchers believe that this built-in quick learning response helps us avoid being poisoned.[18] I used this very research knowledge to help some of my clients gain some temporary control over their constant cravings. My client Monica is one example (**warning:** this case study is not for the faint of heart):

> Monica was undergoing psychotherapy because, as she put it, "My whole life is falling apart." An outside observer probably would have agreed that Monica's life was in disarray. Her husband had admitted to an extramarital affair and had asked her for a divorce so he could move in with his girlfriend. The company where Monica worked was merging with a larger firm, and no one knew which positions would be eliminated. If marital and job crises weren't enough, Monica's mother had also been recently admitted to the hospital.
>
> Clearly, Monica was under considerable life stress. She was also binge-eating on potato chips. She'd gnaw away on at least three large bags a day, and not surprisingly, her weight was rapidly increasing.
>
> "I can't help it!" Monica would protest when I'd ask her about her eating. "My doctor says my blood pressure is up, and I know I need to lay off the salt and high-fat stuff. I can't wear any of my clothes anymore, and it's the worse timing because I need to look polished and professional at work if I'm going to survive this merger. Help me stop bingeing on these damned chips!"
>
> Monica's pleadings and facial expressions reminded me of a prisoner or a caged animal begging for mercy. She felt trapped, controlled by her appetite as if someone else's hands were buying and eating those potato chips.
>
> Of course, Monica—like every one of us—was 100 percent responsible for her eating behavior. No one was putting a gun to her head and forcing her to buy and eat potato chips. I want to make my position on this clear: I'm not advocating that Monica was a victim of any sort. Yet, I also knew that Monica couldn't "hear" any sort of

reasoning about self-responsibility—not until she'd sorted through a lot of confusing and conflicting feelings, anyway. In the meantime, she was destroying herself and needed some crisis intervention.

In cases such as Monica's, where I know that psychotherapy will take some time to affect the appetite, I'll take the temporary measure of inducing a taste aversion. Much like my salmon syndrome, I created a repulsion in Monica toward potato chips.

After warning Monica that my method might create some temporary nausea, we went to work. I put Monica into a hypnotic trance and had her imagine, in complete visual, auditory, olfactory, and taste-sensation detail, a large bowl of potato chips.

I asked her to imagine the sounds of these chips being poured in the bowl, the crackling of the cellophane potato chip bag, and the crunching sound of the chips between her teeth. I asked her to visualize all of the details of the chips and the bowl. She told me she could "see" the salt on the chips' surface, the varied yellow/beige colors, and the twists and shapes of the chips.

Next came the smells, and I asked Monica to fully experience the sensation of smelling the salt, the oil, and the flavors of those chips.

Finally, the taste. Monica imagined the chips' crisp texture against her tongue, the tingling of the salt and the flavor of the potato and oil. We made the image as graphically vivid and real as possible.

Then, I introduced the object that would induce a taste aversion. With Monica still under hypnosis, and with the potato chip image as real as a "virtual reality" experience, I told Monica to envision big, black cockroaches running all throughout the potato chips. Those bugs were scurrying over and contaminating every chip. In fact, she had just eaten a chip that cockroaches had walked upon. She just hadn't noticed those big repulsive bugs until now!

Monica lightly screamed with a start, and her eyes jerked open. She got up and went to the bathroom, because she felt ill. Monica didn't get sick, but she did develop a one-trial aversion toward potato chips. Five months later, as we were concluding our intensive counseling, she still had no desire to eat potato chips.

I've used this method, as a last resort, on many clients, and it's always worked extremely well. You can follow the methods I just described in order to conduct a mini-session with yourself to develop a taste aversion. If you know how to self-hypnotize yourself, the results will be pretty dramatic, as was the case with Monica. Otherwise, do your best to induce a relaxed and uninterrupted state of mind. Conjure up a very real image of your binge food, and then surprise yourself by making the image as grotesque as possible.

As radical as this method may seem, the bottom line is that it really works. Use it as a temporary method, if you like, while you work on the true underlying reasons for your craving.

છે છે છે

WHY DO WE EAT MORE AT BUFFETS AND AT THANKSGIVING?
(The Answer May Surprise You!)

D o you eat more food than normal at all-you-can-eat buffets or salad bars? If you are like most people, the answer is "Yes!" Typically, you go through the buffet line, taking a little of this, a little of that. It all looks so good, and you want just a taste of everything. The trouble is, there are 150 items, and even a tablespoon of each item adds up to a precariously piled plateful of food. Then, you go back for second helpings of your favorite dishes.

What is this phenomenon? Why do we eat more at buffets? Is it an attempt to get our money's worth? Perhaps that's a part of it, but some interesting research points to a more biological basis for buffet-bingeing.

As we discussed in the previous chapter, we have built-in abilities to regulate our nutritional and caloric intake to meet our body's needs. In other words, we intuitively eat enough (usually more than enough!) to keep our body in proper working order.

Along with this intuitive ability, we have an innate drive to consume a variety of food. We instinctively eat different foods so that all of our vitamin, mineral, carbohydrate, protein, and fiber needs are met.

Several studies, performed on both infants and animals, reveal the natural abilities within organisms to select a nutritionally balanced diet. One study allowed infants to eat whatever they chose, and the researchers were pleasantly surprised when the children selected healthful baby foods over "junk" baby foods.[1] The children initially ate sugary sweets, but eventually chose vegetables and fruits.

While analyzing this study, Arthur Halliday, M.D., co-author of *Silent Hunger,* concluded that young children naturally choose healthful foods because they yield the most energy.[2] Another study put laboratory rats in the same free food choice situation, and the results were the same as for human infants. The rats naturally selected a healthful balance of foods.[3]

Variety Equals Quantity

So what does all this have to do with our all-you-can-eat buffet? Well, it seems that all organisms have a drive to seek variety in their diets. The more foods put in front of us, the more we will consume, because of this instinctual drive for nutritional completeness. Our bodies "know" that we'll get vitamin C from one food, and vitamin D from another. We need a full spectrum of vitamins, minerals, and nutritional properties. Back in the cave days, we couldn't pop a Flintstone's vitamin supplement. Instead, we were given the instinct to eat a wide range of foods.

All humans and animals eat more when they are presented with a variety of foods. When laboratory rats were given some chow that had four different smells, their food consumption rose 70 percent within two hours! Other researchers gave rats a "buffet" consisting of potato chips, cheese biscuits, chocolate wafers, and shortbread. A separate control group of rats was given just one choice of food (chips, biscuits, chocolate, etc.) to eat. The buffet-eating rats ate 50 percent more food than the rats with only one food choice.[4]

Human experiments show similar results. The more variety in textures and tastes there is, the more we eat. In one study, two groups of female subjects were told to eat as many sandwiches as they wanted. The first group was offered one type of sandwich; the second group had a variety of different sandwiches available. Not surprisingly, the group with the variety of sandwiches ate 33 percent more than the other group.[5]

Flavor variety can also trigger overeating (for example, we want to "test" all the flavors in a box of assorted chocolates or in a bowl of jelly beans). Researchers studied this phenomenon in an experiment using both male and female subjects. The researchers told the subjects they were conducting a taste test for yogurt flavors (the group members didn't realize the amount of their yogurt consumption was also being monitored). At first, the subjects were given one flavor of yogurt. Thirty minutes later, the subjects were given four flavors of yogurt from which to choose. Even though their hunger was satiated after the first episode of eating, the yogurt varieties stimulated their hunger, and they consumed 33 percent more food at the second sitting![6]

Variety vs. Monotony

If variety stimulates eating, is the reverse also true? Does a monotonous diet lead to less food consumption? The answer appears to be "Yes." Many studies show that animals and humans eat less when they are given a limited choice of foods to eat. Even if you had the option of eating as much of your favorite food as you wanted, you would eat less food than if you were given a six-course meal.

Researchers believe that liquid diets lead to weight loss because the monotony suppresses the appetite. I believe that "food-combining" diets (such as the one made famous in Harvey Diamond's book, *Fit for Life,*) work on the same monotony principle. These diets prohibit the eating of carbohydrates and proteins in the same meal, based on the belief that the body digests each food differently. However, these types of diets probably have less to do with digestion than they do with the amount of food, calories, and fat grams consumed. If you limit the type of food at each meal, you automatically eat less. If you eat less, you lose weight.[7]

Favorite Foods

As I've mentioned previously, the instinct to seek out nutritional variety is more powerful than the drive to eat our preferred foods. If you're like most people, you have a favorite food. Still, you wouldn't want to be limited to eating *only* that food. After a while, you'd get sick of just eating chocolate cake. Or pizza. Or whatever your all-time favorite happens to be. You'd naturally crave something else to eat.

We become "satiated" or satisfied once we've eaten enough of one type of food. Even though it's our favorite, we'll stop eating it if an alternative food is put in front of us. Let's say you're at a restaurant eating your absolute favorite meal, steak. It's cooked just right, exactly the way you like it. And it's a biggie, too—a two-pounder! Then, the waiter delivers a basket of garlic bread. Here's the question: Do you save the remaining room in your stomach for the steak (after all, you absolutely love it, and it's very expensive at that) or do you switch to garlic bread (which is free) and reduce the amount of stomach space available to eat steak?

Without a doubt, you would eat some bread, or salad, or something else in addition to the steak. It's only natural!

Animal studies, both in the laboratory and in the wild, reveal the same phenomenon. The animals were first given their single favorite food, which they wolfed down (so to speak). Then—with that food still readily available—the researchers placed a second, less tasty, food in front of the animals.

Right away, the animals stopped eating their favorite food and ate the less-flavorful secondary food. This research has been replicated many times with similar results.[8]

In another study, noted researcher Paul Rozin fed rats a diet rich in all the essential nutrients except for one: thiamine, also known as vitamin B-1. The rats were allowed to eat as much as they wanted, but they remained deficient in this essential nutrient.

Rozin then placed two large dishes of food in front of the vitamin-deficient rats, and gave them complete freedom to choose between the two foods. The two dishes of food contained identical ingredients, seasonings, and textures. The only difference between the two dishes was that one contained vitamin B-1, and the other did not.

In an amazing demonstration of nature's ability to self-regulate nutrition, the vitamin-deficient rats devoured the vitamin-fortified food and almost none of the vitamin-free food. Some of the rats even turned the vitamin-free food bowls upside down, a behavior that is common when rats don't care for a food. Even after their vitamin needs were replenished, the rats continued to show an aversion toward the vitamin-free version of their food. Other researchers who have studied and replicated Rozin's experiments conclude that rats learn to associate vitamin-deficient food with their bodies being nutritionally deprived. Rats also learn to pair vitamin-enriched food with their bodies being nutritionally fortified.[9]

Could it be that rats are exquisitely sensitive to their body's energy levels, and that being vitamin-deprived is as much an aversive experience as being shocked or hurt? How else were the rats able to distinguish otherwise identical foods, since you can't taste vitamins? It must have been that the rats were tuned in to their bodily reactions to proper nutrients. Hmm…I think we can learn something from these rats, don't you?

The All-You-Can-Eat Restaurant

In Southern California, where I live, there are two types of all-you-can-eat restaurants. The first type is the "soup-and-salad bar" restaurant. For around ten dollars, you can eat as much salad, soup, bread, and muffins as you like. You walk into one of these huge restaurants, and you are instantly confronted with 50 different varieties of chopped vegetables, as well as salad toppings ranging from sunflower seeds to huge home-style croutons. You get to choose from ten different salad dressings, all of them appealing to the eye and the taste buds. Then there are the 12 pasta salads, the seafood salad, the pre-made Caesar salad, and Chinese chicken salad. And that's just the first half of the restaurant!

Next, you walk past hot serving kitchens offering freshly baked biscuits and breads. Of course, there's also a variety of bread spreads, such as whipped honey-butter or fresh boysenberry jam. But wait! We haven't even gotten to the soups yet! Chili, navy bean, New England clam chowder, chicken noodle, and creamy broccoli cheese soups—how can you decide?

The second type of all-you-can-eat restaurant exists in virtually every city in America. Maybe there's one near your home. When I lived in Nashville, Tennessee, where I was program director of an all-women psychiatric hospital, there were several buffets from which to choose.

The typical all-you-can-eat restaurant is virtually the opposite of the soup-and-salad buffet. Whereas the salad buffet is a dazzling display of greens, the all-you-can-eat variety is an acre of various "browns." Most everything at this type of restaurant is breaded, fried, and browned. I can rarely identify what food is being served because it's so well disguised by the frying process. In fact, sometimes you actually have to read the little placard descriptions of each food before you know what you're spooning onto your plate. Otherwise, you might eat a browned "surprise," and discover—too late—that you've got your least-favorite food in your mouth!

There are three principal reasons why we overeat at these buffets:

1. *Variety increases our appetite physically, emotionally, and mentally.* As we've seen, animals and humans eat up to 70 percent more food when presented with a variety. Part of this is an insulin reaction, part of it an emotional response of "Goodie, goodie! Look at all the fun and exciting foods!"

There are novelty dishes served at buffets that you want to try just because they're foods not commonly offered in other restaurants or those which you wouldn't ordinarily cook for yourself at home.

Another part of buffet bingeing is mentally based. There is an intellectual interest in testing each type of food, to learn more about one's own self. You are testing yourself when you taste-test each food, learning about your likes and dislikes.

2. *There's a desire to get your money's worth.* When I go to a salad bar, it's difficult for me to justify spending $10 for one plate of lettuce. I know that the food I'm eating cost the restaurant $2, tops. This is where the mental bargaining game begins: "I'm stuffed, but I don't feel like I ate enough food to justify the money I spent." Then the other side of your logic kicks in: "Who cares how much it costs? If I overeat, I'll regret it later."

   Part of this mental game stems from the very name, "All You Can Eat." That name almost signals a command, or a challenge, to eat until you're stuffed. Maybe that's why some newer buffet restaurants have adopted the alternative slogan, "All You *Care* to Eat." This implies that the restaurant-goer has an option to say, "No, thanks, I don't care to eat another serving."

3. *There are childlike fears about not getting enough to eat.* When we were children, the amount of food doled out to us at meals was controlled by adults. As such, many people carry around leftover fears from childhood that, "I won't get enough to eat," or "I better hurry and eat this food before Mommy clears away the food from the table," or "If I don't clean my plate, I'll get in trouble."

   One of my clients, Maria, came from a large family with ten brothers and sisters. Growing up, the children competed for food at the dinner table. Maria's older brothers shoved and pushed to get the largest helpings of meat, potatoes, and bread. Maria learned young to hoard and stuff food—in her case, it was a matter of survival!

As an adult, these feelings persisted, and Maria would hurriedly consume as much food as possible. Deep down, she still carried the anxiety that her brothers would eat all the food and leave her frustrated and hungry. Not surprisingly, Maria's favorite type of restaurants were the all-you-can-eat variety. Even then, Maria's anxieties weren't quelled by the boundless varieties of available food.

Maria was fortunate, though. Once she exposed her childhood anxieties about getting enough food to eat, she was able to release them. After discussing her fears with me, she instantly saw how illogical it was to carry those fears into adulthood. After all, she and her husband were financially secure. The reality was that Maria could take her time eating, because no one was competing with her at the dining table.

Seven Tips for Avoiding Buffet Binges

Buffet binges and Thanksgiving-Day overeating are such commonplace occurrences that many have accepted them as facts of life. Of course, some compulsive overeaters eat like it was Thanksgiving every single day. They always get up from the table—at every meal—feeling stuffed until their stomach hurts. This feels uncomfortable in a sense, but at the same time the stuffed feeling is somehow nurturing. It's a much safer alternative than facing the underlying feelings or the ramifications of making major life changes. Those are daunting.

I was feeling hungry, and knew it meant I was running from an uncomfortable feeling. I had been having some money problems and had been praying for solutions and guidance. When the answers came, I didn't want to accept them because change is scary—scary for everyone, including myself.

It was one of the times when I'd felt insecure. That always happens when you push yourself to the next level above your comfort zone. Here are the steps I used, and which I recommend, to overcome emotional eating, especially at buffets:

1. *Don't go to a buffet in the first place.* It's a set-up for frustration and feelings of failure. Ask yourself, "Why do I want to go to a buffet at all?" Sometimes, it's a thinly disguised attempt to rationalize overeating. After all, no one *needs* to go to an all-you-can-eat restaurant. We choose to go because we believe such restaurants are fun or are good deals. But, in reality, are restaurants where third helpings are encouraged really fun, or are they just setting you up to feel guilty and uncomfortable afterwards?

2. *Look over the entire buffet before choosing what to eat.* Has this ever happened to you?: You fill your buffet plate with food that you kind of like, that you figure is good for you, and then you happen upon the *really* good food? Your plate is already piled high, but since you don't want to pass up what you want most, you load that food onto your plate, too! Since this invariably happens, why not take evasive action and look over the entire buffet before you put any food on your plate? Walk into that all-you-can-eat restaurant and act like you own the place! Look at each and every dish offered, and ask yourself, "Is this something I can live without, or do I truly want to try it?"

3. *Choose just six foods from the buffet that you want to eat.* Even if you are confronted with a wide variety of foods, you can limit the variety by deciding to eat only a limited number of them. Doing so will reduce the excitement associated with binge-eating on a variety of foods.

4. *Relax and eat slowly.* Much of buffet bingeing comes from an emotional response that says, "I'll never be able to eat this much again!" When we slow down, take deep breaths and relax, we realize that no one is going to take the food from us. No one is going to punish us for eating too much or too quickly. We are adults, and we are in charge. So take a deep breath, and take the time to really enjoy each food on your plate. When you enjoy the taste sensations, you automatically slow down the eating process. And that ensures that you will eat much less.

5. *Drink a large glass of a no-calorie beverage with your meal.* It's always true: if you fill your stomach with water, tea, or diet cola, you'll have less room for food. At all-you-can-eat buffets, this idea makes more sense than ever. Yet, many people avoid drinking a beverage because they want to "save" room for the food they have paid for. You won't make that mistake, will you?

6. *At all-you-can-eat buffets, avoid drinking alcohol.* Alcohol is high in calories, releases inhibitions and, therefore, encourages binge-eating, so avoid wine, beer, and cocktails. Alcohol also slows metabolic digestion of food and beverages, thereby making the calories you've ingested harder to burn off.

7. *No third helpings.* I'm tempted to say, "No second helpings," but that's unrealistic. Instead, when you go to a buffet, a smart eater follows this strategy: Look over the entire buffet, pick out six favorites and limit your choices to those items, go back for second helpings on your absolute favorites, and do not eat third helpings, no matter what.

Thanksgiving Survival Skills

Going home for the holidays doesn't have to be fattening, but for thousands of people, "overeating" and "Thanksgiving" are synonymous.

It happens every year when Judy, a 38-year-old bank manager from Seattle, arrives at her parents' Cincinnati home for her annual one-week holiday visit. "I instantly feel like a gangly, know-nothing little girl," says Judy. "Mom's always telling me to eat, eat! Dad pressures me to settle down and get married." By the time Judy returns to Seattle, her self-confidence is usually shaken, and her weight is up by ten pounds.

Millions of people "go home again" each holiday season, but most family reunions bear little resemblance to the warm family embraces portrayed in the closing scene of the movie, *It's a Wonderful Life*. The strong emotions brought on by spending holidays with relatives encourages some people to overeat.

Many people associate food with holidays. Childhood memories of feeling loved, safe, and happy intertwine with thoughts of Christmas cookies, Passover treats, or Thanksgiving feasts. As adults we turn to those foods for comfort, especially when holiday get-togethers get on our nerves.

As children, we weren't as aware of our relatives during the holidays, because we focused on playing and gifts. But as adults, we become painfully conscious of Uncle Ralph getting tipsy, Aunt Sally's nosy questions, or Cousin Barbara's grating, high-pitched voice. It's uncomfortable to acknowledge that our holiday is less than perfect, so we overeat to comfort ourselves.

Holidays are often filled with unrealistic expectations that lead to disappointment. We may expect holidays to be similar to the ones we experienced as children and dream of being showered with gifts, attention, and love. It's a real letdown when the holiday is mundane or filled with family problems.

Unfortunately, our body never takes a holiday from turning the fat that we eat into body fat. Every year, the average American gains *seven* pounds between Thanksgiving and New Year's Day. This yo-yo weight gain is both unhealthful and frustrating for anyone who has worked hard to stay fit throughout the year. This year, why not take steps to avoid "The Holiday Seven" in the first place? Here are some strategies to help you avoid overeating, *without* sacrificing delicious family traditions!

✦ A major reason people overeat at family gatherings is because old childhood feelings are stirred up, making us feel like awkward, helpless little kids. To combat this tendency, I recommend bringing an "adulthood anchor" to your family's home (unless, of course, the family is coming to *your* home). An adulthood anchor is anything you can look at privately to remind yourself of the competent, grown-up individual you really are. Examples of anchors to bring along include a favorite book, some office work, your business card, your most recent paycheck, or even a college textbook.

✦ It's not a good idea to either publicly confront your irritating relatives, or to stuff your unpleasant feelings by eating food (what I call "fattening feelings"). Instead, get up and excuse yourself from any troubling situations. Go to a private place, such as the rest room or a bedroom. Take a few moments to breathe deeply, and remind yourself that you'll soon be home in your own environment.

There are three ways to combat these irritating fattening feelings when they crop up. First, admit your feelings to yourself instead of fighting or ignoring them. Second, help the troubling emotions subside by either talking about them with a person who's nonjudgmental and a good listener, by writing your feelings in a personal journal, or by going for a walk and talking to yourself about your feelings. Third, don't overeat to compensate for your fattening feelings—that will only make you feel worse!

+ If you feel strongly opposed to a relative's behavior, talk to him or her out of earshot of the rest of the family to avoid additional strife. If you've been drinking, wait until you are both sober before having any kind of serious discussion. You cannot reason with an intoxicated person.

If you are cooking the holiday meal yourself, you're probably aware of the perils of kitchen nibbling. Pre-dinner and post-dinner nibbling can easily double or even triple your consumption of calories and fat grams. We all know that there is a big difference between merely *tasting* a recipe to test its flavor, and *eating* it because the cook is hungry. For that reason, here are four tips for smart cooks to avoid pre-meal overeating:

1. Chew on gum, or suck on a hard candy, while you are cooking. If your mouth is full, you are less apt to engage in absent-minded nibbling.

2. Keep a large glass of a calorie-free beverage such as water, iced tea, or diet soda next to you while you're cooking.

3. Play relaxing background music in the kitchen. Sometimes, jangled nerves and stress lead to overeating. You can avoid nervous nibbling by listening to soothing classical music.

4. Be sure to eat *before* cooking your holiday meal. Many people skip meals before holiday feasts "to save their appetites." But the result of meal-skipping is a hungry cook who overeats in the kitchen!

Even though you may be away from home, stick to your normal exercise routines. The exercise will help raise your energy level while also making you feel more at peace with yourself, thus preventing you from overeating.

The best response to family members who insist that you should "eat more!" is to tell them: "I'm so full that if I eat one more bite, I will explode!" This is a statement no one can argue with. After all, how can you eat more if you are full? Just don't make the mistake of telling family members who are prone to pushiness that you "are on a diet"—unless you want an earful of unsolicited dieting advice!

Some other strategies to avoid overeating:

✦ In some households, you'd be insulting Grandma if you turned down her cooking, even if you've sworn off the high-fat food she's offering you. To avoid unnecessary arguments or hurt feelings, just take a small helping. A few bites of something won't sabotage your health, but it may maintain peace at home. If the food being served is definitely off your eating list—for example, ham or other red meats—you can always resort to the diplomatic practices of mashing the food with your fork, "hiding" it under a biscuit, feeding it to the dog, or walking into the kitchen with your plate and inconspicuously disposing of it.

✦ There is nothing wrong with wanting to relax and enjoy yourself during the holidays. In fact, depriving yourself of traditions and treats can lead to an overeating binge. Limit your treats to those foods only available during the holidays. After all, you can always eat peanuts or chocolates, but pumpkin pie is a special treat for the fall and winter months. A bit of intelligent pre-planning can give you the satisfaction of enjoying traditional holiday treats without gaining weight. Smart substitutions will keep your calories and fat grams down, without leaving you feeling deprived. Here are some examples:

Instead of:	Choose:
Ham, at 350 calories and 28 grams of fat per 3.5 oz.	Turkey, light meat without skin, at 160 calories and 3 grams of fat per 3.5 oz.
Dark turkey meat with skin, at 220 calories and 11.5 gms of fat per 3.5 oz.	Light turkey meat without skin, at 160 calories and 3 grams of fat per 3.5 oz.
Biscuits, at 90 calories and 4.5 fat grams	Wheat roll, at 50 calories and 2 fat grams each
Pecan pie, at 550 calories and 25 fat grams per slice	Pumpkin pie, at 300 calories and 11 fat grams per slice

HOW YOUR PERSONALITY
AFFECTS YOUR WEIGHT

I've always found those one-size-fits-all diets offensive. You know—the ones that tell you exactly what you can and cannot eat? There's this built-in assumption that we're all alike, that everyone can try the same diet and yield similar results. Well, as I'm sure you're aware, we're not all the same!

Since no two people are alike, it's unlikely that one single eating prescription will work for everyone. Yes, we can follow general advice such as eating more fresh fruits and vegetables and consistently exercising. Yet, we all know that such guidelines aren't sufficient to sustain permanent weight loss. The fact is that most people return to unhealthful eating within two years of exhibiting substantial weight loss.

Diets are abandoned for several reasons, as some of my clients' experiences will show:

1. *The recommended menus are too restrictive.* For example, my client Dianna tried a "high-protein" diet, where she was supposed to eat only meat, cheese, eggs, and a few vegetables. Within four days of beginning her diet, Dianna wanted a piece of bread so badly she could barely concentrate on anything else. The amount of food she wanted didn't change; Dianna just craved some nutritional variety.

2. *We rebel against rules.* Like most of us, Brenda hated to be told what to do. Each time she'd begin a new "diet," she felt like a little kid being punished and dominated. When Brenda cheated on her diets, it was her way of exercising control. Each time she'd sneak a candy bar, Brenda was, in essence, sticking out her tongue at the oppressive diet and saying, "Nyah, nyah, you can't tell me what to do!"

3. *Diets don't take our individual lifestyles into consideration.* Harriet travels extensively in her sales job and eats most meals at restaurants. "All the diet clubs want me to eat prepackaged foods, and the diet books all want me to make my own meals," Harriet complained. "Neither option is realistic in conjunction with my job."

4. *Diets don't address our personality differences.* As you'll read in this chapter, your temperament, personality style, and gender all influence your appetite and eating habits. We are multidimensional and complex, and simplistic diets are the equivalent of trying to force a square peg in a round hole.

Was Jack Sprat an Introvert?

Many studies have delved into whether our personality determines our eating behavior. In particular, researchers have studied so-called extroverts and introverts and the differences in their eating styles.

Extroverts, as you probably know, are outgoing, friendly, and talkative. They are the people who are always making telephone calls and who generally dislike being alone. It's estimated that 51 percent of the population are extroverted.

If extroverts are the talkers of the world, introverts are the listeners. They are shy, a little withdrawn, and self-sufficient loners. These are the people who are perfectly happy to be alone.

Neither style is good or bad, right or wrong. But they do appear to correlate to your appetite, eating, and weight. It reminds me of the Mother Goose tale about Jack Sprat and his overweight wife. Remember? *Jack Sprat could eat no fat, his wife could eat no lean...*

Anyway, that verse conjures up the stereotype of the thin, shy, reserved individual and the loud, boisterous, overweight person. Well, it turns out that there are studies explaining why extroverts tend to be heavier than introverts! It appears that:

+ ***Extroverts eat because of external cues***. For example, the clock says "12:00 noon," and the extrovert interprets this as a signal that it's time to eat lunch. Introverts eat due to internal cues—a rumbling stomach, and other signs of hunger.[1]

+ ***Extroverts demand more variety in their diets than introverts.*** A monotonous meal leaves extroverts feeling hungry and dissatisfied, while the introvert walks away with a satiated appetite.[2]

+ ***High-fat foods and highly sweetened foods are more preferred by extroverts than introverts.*** Extroverts report experiencing more intense pleasure while eating, as compared to introverts.[3]

+ ***When an abundance of food is available, extroverts are more likely to gain weight than introverts.*** One study of girls at a summer camp found that girls with an "external" orientation (such as eating in response to the clock instead of hunger) were much more likely to gain weight while at camp, compared to "internally" oriented girls (who eat only in response to hunger).[4]

+ ***Extroverts are more likely to eat just because food is in front of them.*** If there is a plate of cookies in front of you, are you suddenly hungry for those cookies? This is an example of food cravings that are triggered by outside stimuli, rather than food cravings triggered by an emotion. Extroverts have more difficulty resisting readily available food than do introverts.

✦ *Extroverts experience physical reactions at the mere sight of food.* You've probably heard someone say, "I gain weight if I even look at a candy bar." It turns out this may not be far from the truth. The sight of food increases insulin levels much more in externally oriented people than in those who are internally oriented.[5]

Appetite-Reducing Steps for Extroverts

How is all this information relevant to you? If you are an extrovert (like the majority of people), it's important to be aware of how this external orientation can trigger overeating. Extroverts often ignore their gut feelings because they are tuned into cues from the outer world. Here are some strategies for extroverts struggling with an overactive appetite:

1. *Pay attention to internal hunger cues.* As we've discussed previously, it's important not to automatically eat in response to external cues. We can retrain ourselves to become internally oriented to hunger cues. Instead of relying on the clock ("It's noon, so I must eat lunch"), we must rely on our body to tell us when to eat. Reread the steps in Chapter 2 that detail the ways to avoid emotional eating.

2. *Beat the multi-course meal habit.* A nutritionally balanced meal doesn't require a multitude of side dishes. Vegetable, protein, and carbohydrate needs can be met with three to four menu items. Be especially careful around buffets, where the variety may tempt you to overeat (see Chapter 6). As an

extrovert, you are even more vulnerable to buffet bingeing, so you may want to think twice before making restaurant reservations at that new all-you-can-eat establishment. Maybe the temptation is not even worth it.

3. *Minimize your exposure to food stimuli.* Researcher Bernard Lyman, Ph.D., writes, "In externally responsive individuals, the insulin level rises at the sight of food, and this increases hunger. There has been some success treating the obese by minimizing their exposure to food stimuli. Little food is kept in the home, and the individuals are encouraged not to read articles discussing food or food preparation, to avoid food advertisements, and to stay away from supermarkets except to buy needed foods and then in very small quantities. 'Out of sight, out of mind' seems to reduce food intake for some people."[6]

4. *Center yourself before eating.* Give your gut feelings a chance to be heard above the din. I'd love to see extroverts adopt the habit of saying a prayer before mealtime. Before picking up your fork, lower your eyes, take a breath, go inward, and say grace in your own way. Your body will relax, and your inner voice will reward you with valuable guidance and inspired information.

Staying tuned in to gut feelings requires some patience and practice. It takes about 30 days to change habits, so hang in there. You deserve the best, including a free spirit and a light body!

ॐ   ॐ   ॐ

THE INTERPRETATION
OF FOOD CRAVINGS

HOW FOODS CHANGE OUR MOODS

Everything we put in our mouths—whether it's beverages, food, or pills—affects our bodies, energy levels, mind, and moods. The very structure of that food, drink, or drug influences us in many critical ways.

If this sounds like an extreme statement, let me back up. Most people readily accept the idea that food affects work performance and energy levels. For example, few parents would dream of sending their child to school without breakfast, since it's accepted that children need proper nutrition for optimum achievement.

Scientific studies confirm that children perform worse on intellectual and performance tests after skipping even one breakfast.[1] Other studies show that an iron-deficient, protein-deficient[2], or high-fat diet[3] impairs learning and aptitude.

The majority of people acknowledge the role that nutrition plays in athletics. We watch athletes carbohydrate-loading prior to a sporting event, since they know that carbohydrates are crucial to stamina and energy.

Drugs and alcohol, two major mood-alterers, are derived from foods. For example, the drug used to treat manic depression is a sodium compound called *lithium*. That's right—a form of salt eases the extremist forms of depression and anxiety! Alcohol, on the other hand, is produced from fermented fruits and grains. So it's not a stretch to see that other foods can impact one's thinking, energy levels, and emotions. Consider this: when our energy is low, we tend to feel depressed. If we are truly depressed, a low energy level makes us feel even worse.

When our thoughts are scattered or when we're not thinking straight, it's easy to *think our way* into a bad mood. We begin to harbor fears that other people don't like us or that our life is a horrible mess. And these faulty ideas form the core of negative emotions.

Since thoughts and energy are at least partially shaped by nutrition, it follows suit that the foods we eat can change and affect our moods. Every food contains minerals, vitamins, and amino acids that permeate our entire body, and which can affect it in positive or negative ways.

The amino acids in foods are particularly influential, as they can be divided into two categories: psychoactive (mood-altering), or vasoactive (energy-altering). Psychoactive amino acids influence our moods by changing the brain chemistry ("neurotransmitters") in the central nervous system. Vasoactive amino acids affect our energy levels by stimulating or relaxing our blood pressure or heart rate.

Some foods, like some beverages or drugs, are "stronger" than others. They contain more mood-altering or energy-altering properties than do other foods. Those foods will create more intense energy or mood shifts than milder foods.

Tyramine, for example, is a powerful stimulant found naturally in aged cheese, chocolate, pickled foods, soy sauce, vanilla, yogurt, and beer and wine. Tyramine is a strong vasoconstrictor that increases blood pressure. In fact, the stimulant effect of tyramine is so strong that physicians warn their patients who are on antidepressant medication (Monoamine Oxidase, or MAO therapy) to avoid foods with tyramine. The interaction between MAO and tyramine can trigger hypertensive crises. Other studies show that highly sensitive individuals may suffer from migraine headaches brought on by eating foods high in tyramine.[4]

Food Cravings and Sensitivity

As the intensity of food's properties vary, so does an individual's sensitivity to the mood-altering effects of food. Some people are exquisitely sensitive to their own body's chemistry and have intense reactions to alcohol, chocolate, coffee, and sugar. These substances kick them in the head like a shot of morphine.

How sensitive are you to your body's chemistry? Have you noticed any of these reactions in yourself?

+ You feel sluggish after eating a big meal.
+ You feel a little lightheaded after drinking a diet soda.
+ Eating calms your nerves.
+ When you're under stress, you immediately think about what foods or drinks could soothe you.
+ You crave chocolate or salty foods right before your menstrual cycle.
+ You prefer to eat ice cream whenever you're feeling depressed.
+ You feel enveloped in warmth and pleasure when you eat chocolate.
+ You have negative reactions to Chinese food containing MSG.
+ When you want instant energy, you eat a candy bar or drink a caffeinated beverage.

If you answered yes to three or more questions, you show signs of being sensitive to your body chemistry. Sensitive individuals often require less medication for pain, and less anesthesia for operations. They also feel the effects of adrenaline more intensely. For example, following a near-miss with another car, a sensitive individual may feel shaky, as a result of the adrenaline rush, for up to an hour after the incident.

Food Cravings or Food Allergies?

Some researchers see food cravings as a symptom of underlying food allergies. The theory is that those who have allergies metabolize food differently than nonallergic people. Those with allergies exhibit two adverse reactions: they crave the food they are allergic to, and they have psychological reactions after eating the food.

One experiment that has lent credence to this theory was performed by a researcher named David King. He gathered together 30 people who struggled with intense food cravings. King asked each subject to name the foods they craved most, and to reveal their typical emotional reaction to eating that food. He didn't tell the subjects the study's true purpose.

The most commonly named cravings were for wheat, beef, milk, and sugar. King made liquid extracts of each food and placed a few drops under the tongues (one at a time, of course), of each subject. King then asked each person to guess what the food extract was, as well as to describe any resulting emotional reactions. In addition, King put placebo liquids under the subject's tongues at random intervals. (The study was double-blind, meaning that King wasn't aware of which extract or which placebo he was placing in the subject's mouth).

The results were notable. The subjects reported significantly higher emotional reactions, including depression and irritability, when they were given the food they most often craved.[5]

Food's Mood-Altering Properties

I'm sometimes misunderstood when I discuss the mood-altering chemicals in food. Some assume that I'm talking about pesticides or some other foreign ingredients. Therefore, I try to use the term *mood-altering properties*. *Properties* is actually a more accurate word than *chemicals* since the parts of food that influence us include four separate components:

1. *The basic amino-acid structures of the food.* Amino acids are either psychoactive (mood-altering) or vasoactive (energy-altering). Psychoactive amino acids affect the brain's neurotransmitters. Vasoactive amino acids influence blood pressure and pulse rate, and are either vasoconstricting or vasodilating. Amino acids are either stimulating or soothing:

    a. **Stimulating.** The amino acid vasoconstrictors reduce the size of blood vessels, which squeeze the blood and increase the blood pressure. This makes you feel energized. The stimulating psychoactive amino acids increase the production of excitatory neurotransmitters.

    b. **Calming.** The vasodilator amino acids increase the size of the blood vessel, slowing down the flow of blood and reducing blood pressure. The calming psychoactive amino acids increase the production of inhibitory neurotransmitters.

2. *The texture of the food.* Whether it is soft, crunchy, creamy, or chewy.

3. *The inherent properties in the food: fat content, flavor, seasonings, and spices.* The fat content and spiciness of a meal can alter our physical and emotional states. Some spices, such as cinnamon, sugar, or peppermint, are energy-altering on their own.

4. *The smell.* The aromas of foods affect our moods in two ways: by reminding us of past moments associated with the smell, and by molecular structures of the odors that influence our brain's chemistry.

So let's look briefly at each of these four variables. I'll try not to err on either side by being overly simplistic or overly technical (since I don't enjoy reading either type of material myself). Instead,

I'll strive to keep this material relevant, so no one will say, "So what?" or "What did she just say?"

Serotonin: The Energy and Mood Controller

In previous chapters, I've mentioned the brain chemical, serotonin. Over the last 15 years, scientists have identified this liquid brain messenger as essential in controlling sleep, mood, energy levels, food cravings, and PMS symptoms.

Basically, the brain fires electrical impulses that trigger brain chemical reactions which, in turn, impact our bodies. The brain chemicals, called neurotransmitters, regulate our energy, moods, memory, sex drive, and appetite. Neurotransmitters are either excitatory and stimulating, or they are inhibitory or calming. The production of neurotransmitters is affected by things in the environment such as sunlight, stress, and our nutritional diet.

I like to think of serotonin as fuel in the gas tank. Too much fuel, and your engine is flooded and conked-out. Too little fuel, and your engine won't start at all. If we have too little or too much serotonin, we feel cranky, irritable, depressed, or anxious, and hungry for foods such as sweets or carbohydrates. A serotonin deficit feels like a terrible hangover.

Your brain must produce serotonin on a daily basis. You can't store it or save it from the previous day (like your car's gas tank does!). We produce serotonin at night, while we're dreaming. That's right, during the Rapid Eye Movement (REM) state, we're busily producing enough fuel to ensure an even mood and steady energy level for the next day.

Under normal conditions, where we've maintained a reasonable level of life stress, a balanced nutritional diet, and been exposed to sunlight and exercise, we sleep well and wake up feeling refreshed.

If we wake up feeling tired, wondering, "Did I even get any sleep last night?," the culprit behind the lethargy is usually a low gas tank of serotonin. Several factors can trigger low levels of serotonin:

1. *Excessive life stress.* Each person's tolerance of stress is different. What I might consider intolerable, you might take with a grain of salt. What matters is what *you*, truthfully, find stressful. Under stress, we undergo bodily and behavioral changes that deplete serotonin.

2. *Insomnia.* If you don't get sufficient REM sleep, your body doesn't have the opportunity to refuel its serotonin supply.[6] REM sleep is the equivalent of pulling into the gas station; without these pit-stops, your tank will run dry.

3. *Long-term dieting.* Those who are chronic dieters and who have restricted their caloric intake for many years may have lower serotonin levels than "normal" eaters. Studies with rats show that long-term caloric restriction alters and lowers the concentration of serotonin in the brain. In other words, if you've dieted for years, your body may be craving foods (primarily carbohydrates) that will increase the serotonin level.[7]

4. *Low exposure to sunlight.* Have you ever seen a depressed person close their drapes so that their rooms are as dark as their moods? Perhaps you've read or heard that the onset of winter and its cold, dark days can trigger Seasonal Affective Disorder (SAD), a form of depression, in some individuals? Are you aware of the high suicide rates in dreary, rainy parts of the country such as Seattle and Portland? Researchers blame this phenomenon on serotonin. During REM sleep, the body produces serotonin from the body chemical, *melatonin*. Melatonin is produced in response to sunlight exposure. The more sunlight you take in, the more melatonin—and, thus, serotonin—your body is able to produce.
    Sunlight exposure occurs through the eye's iris. People who receive no sunlight exposure due to complete blindness have major serotonin impairments, including chronic

insomnia, circadian (based on a 24-hour cycle) rhythm disorders, and premenstrual syndrome difficulties.

SAD symptoms include carbohydrate cravings, compulsive overeating, and wintertime weight gains. These cravings are an attempt to self-regulate the brain's depleted serotonin.[8] Treatment for SAD involves exposing the individual to full-spectrum light. Those who become depressed during the winter must expose themselves to a home treatment of special light bulbs or a light screen in order to increase their depleted serotonin.

Some researchers believe that people who live in sunny climates exhibit fewer signs of depression than people who inhabit countries with a minimal amount of sunny days per year. What do you think? Have you ever traveled to a sunny locale and felt your mood or energy level change? How did this compare to your moods in an overcast or rainy locale?

5. *Excessive alcohol, chemicals, or drugs.* Some pharmaceutical products are designed to change our energy levels or moods. They do this by affecting the levels of serotonin. Many of the antidepressant medications on the market today, including Prozac and tricyclic antidepressants, make people feel better by altering serotonin's manufacturing cycles (also called uptake and reuptake).

It's very difficult to increase serotonin levels to such a degree that it would negatively impact a person's energy or mood. Yet, many antidepressants do just that. People taking antidepressants normally feel terrific for the first couple of days because their serotonin level is up. But then the medication overdoes it and increases serotonin too much. The person then experiences depressing or hostile feelings.

Other chemicals, including alcohol and Valium, affect serotonin because they lessen the amount of time we spend in REM sleep.[9] The main reason you feel hungover after a drinking binge is that you haven't had enough dreams (despite those crazy dreams you remember from the early morning hours) to satisfy your serotonin-manufacturing needs.

Valium, and other similar tranquilizers, completely inhibit REM sleep. Not only that, but Valium has a "half-life." The day after you take one Valium, there is still one-half a Valium active within you. So when you take another Valium, you now have 1-½ Valiums active within you.

If you remember the movie or book, *I'm Dancing As Fast As I Can,* you recall the craziness associated with Valium withdrawal. Valium users who stop taking the drug "cold turkey" often have hallucinations for one main reason: all those days of inhibited REM sleep are trying to make up for lost time. When you stop taking Valium, your body begins to have dreams—even when you're awake. All those pent-up dreams come rushing forward in a flood of wide-awake hallucinations.

6. *Menstrual cycle and menstrual fluctuations.* Hormonal fluctuations, triggered by the menstrual cycle, deplete serotonin levels. One of the main causes of PMS symptoms is depleted serotonin.[10] This is also one culprit behind those irritating premenstrual cravings for chocolate, potato chips, and ice cream.

7. *Exercise.* The amount of exercise you have during the day, particularly of the aerobic variety, affects serotonin levels. Studies show that aerobic-level exercise significantly increases the amount of serotonin in the brain.[11] Further, it doesn't matter whether you are normally a sedentary person or a regular athlete—your serotonin level increases in response to exercise, no matter what your physical condition.[12]

8. *Type A or Type B personalities.* There is impressive evidence that Type A personalities—those with free-floating anger, who are perpetually trying to beat the clock, and who are hard-

driving workaholics—have lower levels of serotonin than the calmer, more sedate Type B's. Interestingly enough, serotonin increases much more after the Type A engages in some form of physical activity than it does after the Type B exercises. Researchers conclude that Type A's who exercise (thus, keeping their serotonin levels sufficiently high) are able to suppress feelings of fatigue and endure higher levels of exertion for longer periods of time.[13]

9. *Our present body weight*. One study compared the levels of serotonin in obese individuals with lean individuals. The findings: serotonin was significantly lower in obese individuals than in lean individuals. Whether obesity is a cause or effect of low serotonin is open to speculation at this point.[14]

How Food Impacts Serotonin

Clearly, there are a number of environmental, lifestyle, and personality factors influencing the production of serotonin. Still, *one of the primary factors affecting serotonin production and serotonin levels is the food we eat*.

Just as drugs and alcohol block or encourage serotonin's production, so do the molecular components of food. In particular, serotonin levels are affected by the vitamins, amino acids, and nutritional categories that form the core structure of food. Each food group is individually addressed in Chapters 11 through 21, so for now we'll look at this topic in general.

VITAMINS

Vitamin B-6 (also known as *pyridoxine)* is necessary for serotonin production, as well as for metabolizing tryptophan.[15] When we're deficient in vitamin B-6, our serotonin levels become low.[16] Vitamin B-6 deficiencies, and thus serotonin deficiencies, result in:

- fatigue,
- the inability to exercise vigorously[17],
- irritability,
- depression, and
- pain, including headaches, carpal tunnel syndrome and PMS[18].

Conversely, these symptoms dissipate or even disappear with B-6 supplementation. One study concluded that 100 milligrams (mg) daily of vitamin B-6 was sufficient for keeping serotonin at optimum levels.[19] Doctors caution against taking more than 200 mg a day; vitamin B-6 can be toxic at such levels if taken for several months.[20]

We would have to eat a lot of food to get 100 mg of vitamin B-6, though. Even the foods highest in this vitamin contain less than 1 mg per serving. Foods high in vitamin B-6 include:

- avocados (the highest, with .85 mg in a medium avocado),
- bananas,
- chicken,
- green peas,
- potatoes,
- walnuts, and
- wheat germ.

Since it's difficult to eat sufficient Vitamin B-6 in order to keep serotonin levels high, it's possible that many of us who don't take a supplement are B-6-depleted. This could lead to food cravings as the body attempts to increase the B-6 and serotonin supply.

Any time serotonin is low, the body will try to correct this deficiency. All organisms are geared toward homeostasis, that is, the state where the body is comfortable and adequately nourished. When any essential element is low, the body tries to adjust it. In the case of serotonin deficits, the adjustment comes in the form of food cravings. Sometimes these cravings are for the foods named above, which contain B-6. But many other foods encourage serotonin production, and that's why our cravings are so diverse, as you'll read.

AMINO ACIDS

If you've been to a gym or a health-food store in the last ten years, you've undoubtedly seen amino acid supplements. You may also remember the L-tryptophan scandal in the late 1980s. Several people died after taking this supplement, and the Center for Disease Control (CDC) took immediate action and banned its sale. An investigation later revealed that a Japanese vitamin packager's unsanitary practices led to the fatal poisonings. Rather than ban the Japanese producer from doing business in the U.S., the CDC simply removed L-tryptophan from the market.

The poisonings were front-page news; however, when the actual reason for the deaths was revealed, it was usually reported on back pages of the newspapers. As a result, many consumers were left with the mistaken impression that tryptophan itself was inherently poisonous. In fact, the poison in those pills came from contamination, including vermin waste and other sanitation violations on the part of the manufacturer.

Prior to the ban of L-tryptophan, I, along with many medical doctors, psychologists, and hospitals, was using the amino acid in treating such disorders as alcoholism, anxiety, depression, drug abuse, eating disorders, insomnia, and premenstrual syndrome. These conditions are all a function of serotonin levels, and the L-tryptophan supplements seemed to help alleviate many symptoms.

TRYPTOPHAN IN FOOD

Tryptophan (the L- or the D- in front of the name just signifies whether the amino acid is synthetic or organic, and really is an inconsequential term) is a precursor of serotonin. This means that it is a catalyst, or instrumental agent, responsible for making serotonin.

Remember the analogy of serotonin to gasoline?—how we need enough "fuel" for the car (our body) to run, but not so much gasoline to flood the engine? Well, think of tryptophan as the fossil fuel from which gasoline is made.

After we eat tryptophan, in pill or the proper food form, and it crosses our blood-brain barrier (see "Protein" section, page 107), serotonin is produced. The result: we feel great!

Here's a list of the foods highest in tryptophan. Are any of these foods those that you commonly crave?

FOODS HIGH IN TRYPTOPHAN

Food	Mg of Tryptophan
Dairy Products:	
Cottage cheese, 1 cup, 1% fat	312
Cottage cheese, 1 cup, 2% fat	346
Ice cream, 1 cup vanilla	100
Milk, 1 cup, low-fat or whole	113
Milk, 1 cup, nonfat	118
Parmesan cheese, 1 ounce	137
Swiss cheese, 1 ounce	114
Fish and Shellfish *(all are cooked, 3.5-ounce portions):*	
Bass	231
Cod	260
Haddock	196
Halibut	315
Lobster	152
Mackerel	283
Salmon	270
Shrimp	242
Tuna	247

Beef (all are cooked portions):

Hamburger, 1 patty, 85 grams, lean	303
Porterhouse steak, 100 grams, lean	297
Round steak, top portion, 111 grams, lean	504
Sirloin steak, 125 grams, lean	373
T-bone steak, 95 grams, lean	281

Lamb (all are cooked portions):

Blade chop, one lean, 93 grams	329
Loin chop, 3.5 oz.	298
Rib chop, lean, 3.5 oz.	263

Pork (all are cooked portions):

Bacon, Canadian, 63 grams (approx. 3 slices)	180
Bacon, cured, 5 slices (6 grams each)	95
Blade steak, 3.5 oz.	323
Ham, 3.5 oz.	427
Loin chop, 3.5 oz.	382
Sausage, 5 links (13 grams each)	100
Sausage, 2 patties (27 grams each)	84
Spare ribs, 6 medium (90 grams total)	198
Tenderloin, 3.5 oz.	398

Poultry (all are cooked portions):

Chicken breast, ½ (86 grams), without skin	311
Chicken drumstick, 2 (88 grams total), without skin	290
Chicken thighs, 2 (102 grams total), without skin	316
Duck, 100 grams (3.5 oz.), without skin	327
Turkey light meat, 100 grams (3.5 oz.), without skin	340
Turkey dark meat, 100 grams (3.5 oz.), without skin	325

Nuts:

Cashews, roasted (50 grams), 20-25 nuts	215
Mixed nuts (50 grams)	236
Peanuts, roasted without skin (50 grams)	196
Pumpkin seeds (50 grams)	261
Sesame seeds (50 grams)	241
Sunflower seeds (50 grams)	180

It's an interesting list, isn't it? I've only listed foods high in tryptophan, and you may notice that bananas are not on the list. Bananas, like turkey, are reputed to be high in tryptophan. In truth, one medium banana contains only 14 mg of tryptophan, and turkey has the same tryptophan levels as chicken.

PROTEIN

Protein, which is found in meat, fish, and fowl, is made almost entirely of amino acids. So, protein contains a lot of tryptophan. Yet, surprisingly, protein doesn't create a lot of serotonin. That's because all of the other amino acids in protein compete with the tryptophan. To get inside the brain, in order to make serotonin, amino acids have to pass through a huge barrier, called a "blood brain barrier." This requires a lot of strength and power.

When a lot of different amino acids are all competing to get across the brain's barrier, it's like a big gang fight! All the amino acids get pretty beat up, and by the time they get to the barrier, they're too pooped to get across. So when we eat an amino acid-rich food, such as beef, poultry, or fish, we really won't get much of a tryptophan, or serotonin, boost.

CARBOHYDRATES

Compared to protein, carbohydrates contain little tryptophan. That doesn't matter, however. When we eat a meal containing carbohydrates, the angry gang of competing amino acids aren't around to bully or weaken the tryptophan that it does contain.

When we eat carbohydrates, our body secretes insulin. The insulin is like some cool kid who offers to take all the gang members for a ride downtown in his hot new car. Tryptophan isn't invited along, but that's okay; he'd rather stay alone and go to the brain. So insulin "distracts" the bully amino acids by transporting them to the skeleton. That leaves our hero, tryptophan, free to travel to the brain!

Following a high-carbohydrate meal, one which is protein-free, most people feel calm, relaxed, or even tired. This is from the rush of tryptophan to the brain, and the resulting increase in serotonin.[21] When we eat protein-free junk food, such as sweets or snacks, we experience an energy crash. We've referred to this experience as "blood sugar fluctuations" in the past; however, scientists today credit increased serotonin for the post-candy energy crunch.[22]

Craving-Reducing Pills?

New drugs, already sold in Europe and coming soon to American pharmacies, reduce carbohydrate and fat cravings by increasing serotonin. Initial trials with *fenfluramine* and *dexfenfluramine,* known as "serotoninergic agents," reduced carbohydrate cravings by 40 to 55 percent, and fat cravings by 67 percent. The drugs slowed the pace at which the stomach emptied; fat cravings were reduced because the stomach felt full longer.[23]

The long-term safety of these drugs is currently being examined, and so far, so good. Still, some scientists wonder about the wisdom of messing with the brain. Is it worth risking brain damage in order to live craving-free? Undoubtedly, many people would answer, "You bet it's worth it!"

Yet, I still believe in taking a more natural approach. Instead of masking the cravings, why not heal them? Low serotonin, as we've seen, is a product of a stressed-out lifestyle. Insomnia, worry, lack of exercise, and excessive alcohol or caffeine all lower the serotonin level. Instead of adding one more chemical to the equation, why not adjust the lifestyle so that serotonin production is naturally adequate?

I'm also a little concerned that some Americans are waiting for a miracle diet pill to be widely available, seeing this as the cure-all they've been seeking. Many television news shows have teased the public into believing a "fat pill" is on its way. In reality, this medication will only be available in a limited manner. A medical doctor will have to determine a medical necessity for taking the pill, and then the patient will need continual monitoring. The medication, in most instances, won't be covered by health insurance and will likely be quite expensive. In other words, it won't be like going to the drug store and buying a diet pill over the counter.

We are not meant to live our lives dependent upon prescription medication. Our brains were created healthy and whole, and we've got the ability to produce enough serotonin to eradicate any constant craving. Instead of focusing on masking the symptoms of a stressed-out life, why not take whatever small steps are possible to de-stress our lives?

How Food Impacts Other Neurotransmitters

Serotonin is the boss in the brain, as far as neurotransmitters that affect mood and energy levels are concerned. However, there are other brain chemicals that have some say-so about how wide-awake or how tired we feel. The brain chemicals that regulate energy include norepinephrine, epinephrine, noradrenaline, and acetylcholine.

These other neurotransmitters are also affected by the foods we eat. Each brain chemical, or neurotransmitter, is created out of a specific food source, also known as a "precursor." Here are the precursors for these energy-altering brain chemicals:

Neurotransmitter	Precursor Amino Acids/Vitamins
Norepinephrine and Epinephrine	Tyrosine
Noradrenaline	Tyramine
Acetylcholine	Choline/Lecithin

Those precursors are derived from foods. Here is a list of the foods containing high amounts of the precursors for the neuro-transmitters. If you've been craving any of these foods, it's probably because you're overly tired and crave an increase in your energy level. One study found that obese individuals have lower-than-normal levels of norepinephrine, as well as low serotonin.[24] With these two important energy regulators low, obese persons are more likely to crave carbohydrates, as well as the foods below, those which trigger norepinephrine production.

Tyrosine-high and tyramine-high foods:

+ Avocados and bananas
+ Cereals, especially Cheerios, Life, oat flakes and oatmeal, and wheat germ
+ Cashews and peanuts
+ Dairy products, especially cheddar cheese, cottage cheese and cream cheese; ice cream and ice milk
+ Eggs
+ Figs and sulfur-dried fruits
+ Meat, especially liver, sausage, and tuna fish
+ Pickled foods, including pickles, pickled herring, and sauerkraut
+ Soy derivatives, including lecithin and soy sauce
+ Wine and beer

Choline-high foods:
- Eggs
- Flour, especially wheat and soybeans
- Beef and lamb
- High-fat dairy products
- Rice
- Cashews

By craving and eating these foods, you are attempting to perk yourself up. Craving these foods is no different than craving an espresso or other highly caffeinated food. Remember, food cravings are an unconscious desire to feel better, either through getting more energy or by receiving more comfort and pleasure. We intuitively know which foods will achieve our desired ends.

The Texture of Food

The second component of food cravings has to do with the physical makeup of the food. Is it crunchy? Is it smooth? Is it creamy? Is it chunky? Your mouth puts in special orders for specific food textures according to the result, or level of satisfaction, that is desired.

Each variation in food texture signifies a different underlying emotional desire. Those who crave crunchy foods are seeking a source of relief from the two core FATS feelings, Anger and Tension. Variations of these emotions, leading to crunchy food cravings, include frustration, anger, stress, or resentment.

Those who crave creamier, smoother-textured foods are struggling with the other two FATS feelings, Fear or Shame, and are seeking comfort and reassurance. Variations of these feelings include anxiety, embarrassment, and insecurity.

Chewy cravings (such as those for caramel candy or a cheesy pizza) signal a combination of feelings. These could include Fear mixed with Anger (for example, my client Barbara was angry with her boss for ordering her to give a speech at the upcoming convention), or Tension mixed with Shame (my client Sharon was uptight because she doubted her ability to create a new advertising campaign for her client).

THE MEANING OF FOOD TEXTURES

Crunchy food cravings = Hard emotions: These are the emotions that are outwardly directed, as if you want to scream or get back at someone who has hurt you. These feelings include Anger, Bitterness, Frustration, Resentment, Stress, and Tension. *The core FATS feelings behind crunchy food cravings are Anger and Tension.*

Soft or creamy food cravings = Soft emotions: These are the emotions that are inwardly directed. You are angry at yourself (justifiably or not), or you have a deep longing for comfort and reassurance. These feelings include Anxiety, Betrayal, Depression, Embarrassment, Fear, Grief, Insecurity, Regret, Sadness, Self-doubt, and Shame. *The core FATS feelings behind soft or creamy food cravings are Fear and Shame.*

Chewy food cravings = Combination emotions: These are a combination of hard and soft emotions—in other words, Fear or Shame mixed with Anger or Tension. *A combination of one hard (Anger or Tension) and one soft (Fear or Shame) FATS feeling are behind chewy food cravings.*

The Inherent Properties in Food

The third factor involved in food-craving analysis is the physical makeup of the food you are hungry for. I won't go into too many details here since later on in the book, I've devoted a chapter to each food group. Those chapters are devoted to analyzing the craving-producing properties of each food.

In general, some inherent properties in food that affect mood and energy are:

1. *Its fat content*. High-fat cravings for foods such as cheese-burgers, soft french fries, rich milk shakes, and the like signal the first FATS feeling: Fear. The fears can vary, but generally they have to do with a hesitance to face something. This could mean confronting something you don't like in your life, or coming to the realization that you need to make some changes. That fear feels like emptiness, so the Fat Craver tries to eradicate the feeling by maintaining a full stomach. Fat fills up the stomach like nothing else! It essentially clogs the drains of the stomach, slowing down digestion and the emptying of gastric juices.

2. *Its flavor*. Different flavors create different moods and energy levels. To analyze a craving, you need to look at the feeling produced by each flavor. For example, peppermint boosts energy; chocolate boosts production of a drug that feels like love; and hot and spicy food creates feelings of excitement, energy, and a "feeling no pain" mindset.

The Smell of Food

The human capacity to detect smell is phenomenal. We can detect a microscopic change in the smell of our environment and are nearly as sensitive as smoke alarms in detecting smoky odors.[25]

Our sense of smell definitely affects our appetite and food cravings. You've probably experienced a blunted appetite when your nose is clogged during a head cold. Part of the pleasure of eating is the enjoyment of the delicate wafts of enticing aromas. It's no accident that realtors claim they can sell a house quicker if bread or cookies are baking during sales expeditions!

Biologists have theorized that we humans developed this keen sense of smell to survive in the wild. Deep in our subconscious, we actually have the ability to smell the difference between poisonous and edible food.

In our modern lives, smell affects appetite in two ways:

1. *By the memories it conjures up.* Our sense of smell is directly linked to our memory banks. We'll smell a cologne and be transported back to a lost-love experience. We smell orange blossoms and re-experience a wedding. We smell vinegar and relive the Easter egg-dyeing times of our childhood. There's a lot of evidence that our olfactory sense—our sense of smell—is more directly tied to our memory banks than any other sense.[26]

2. *By the psychoactive chemicals we ingest through smelling.* Foods in the nut group—including coffee, chocolate, and all nuts—give off an odor called *pyrazine*. Pyrazine triggers the pleasure center of the brain, stimulating the production of many feel-good chemicals. This mood-altering chemical reaches our brain through our olfactory senses—that is, through our noses. That's one of the reasons why the smell of ground coffee or mixed nuts makes us feel so good when we first open the can.[27]

Chicago neurologist and psychiatrist, Dr. Alan Hirsch, has made a career of studying the effects of smells on human behavior and emotions. He explains the link this way, "Of all the human senses, the olfactory sense (of smell) has the greatest impact on the emotions because the olfactory sensory apparatus is intertwined with the limbic system—the part of the brain associated with emotions." Among Hirsch's findings:

✦ The smell of vanilla makes people feel happier and more relaxed.

✦ Citrus aromas are stimulating.

✦ The smell of green apple, peppermint, and banana led to reduced appetite and weight loss in his patients. The more they smelled these substances, the more weight they lost, and the average weight-loss was 2.1 percent of body fat.

✦ Strawberry odors motivate people to exercise.

✦ Men are very aroused by the smell of baked cinnamon buns.[28]

What's interesting to me is that every one of Dr. Hirsh's findings dovetails with my own research, as well as those of other scientists. It makes perfect sense, for example, that the smell of peppermint would correlate with weight loss. Peppermint is a stimulant. If you feel energized, you're less apt to seek out a food that will pep up your energy level. You'll eat less and lose some weight.

SELF-HELP FOR FOOD CRAVINGS

Our appetite was created to operate perfectly, just like the rest of our body and mind. As you've read, food cravings are part of a flawlessly engineered system that functions in a fairly predictable and systematic way.

Those of us who've struggled with weight have assumed that our out-of-control appetites meant that something was wrong with us. After all, overweight people are often accused of being lazy or lacking will power. Yet, there's nothing defective about food cravings; they are a natural response to a high-stress lifestyle and repressed emotions.

When we try to ignore our feelings or burn the candle at both ends (without sufficient fuel), our body responds in the way it was originally programmed at the "factory." We have intense cravings for the food that will correct our stress-depleted brain chemicals. Food cravings are as natural and predictable as a startled reaction to a sudden loud noise.

We've tried diets in the past, hoping to *kill* our appetites. But why would we want to kill a part of ourselves? How does that wish impact our self-esteem? It's as if we're declaring to the universe, "There's a part of me that is bad, defective, and wrong!" It's a form of rejecting one's self. This is an unkind way to treat ourselves, wouldn't you agree? Self-esteem is based upon self-acceptance. Instead of trying to kill your appetite, let's work on healing your appetite.

Here are some step-by-step recommendations for releasing your food cravings:

+ ***Break the automatic eating habit.*** As you've read throughout this book, those with the strongest food cravings are often outer-focused extroverts and Mood Eaters. Extroverts are externally focused, eating because the clock says it's lunchtime and not because their stomach signals hunger. Mood Eaters are running away from the awareness of their uncomfortable feelings. The more they run away, the stronger the food cravings become.

    Mood Eaters know the source of their unhappiness deep down, but have decided that facing these feelings would result in more discomfort. It's an all-or-nothing thinking style that is a hallmark of the addictive personality. (Usually, there are lots of different options for anyone who faces problems square-on. You've probably had this pleasant realization yourself).

    Automatic eating means you eat whenever you have the thought, "I'm hungry." In order to heal the appetite, we've got to allow your food cravings a few minutes to speak their message to you. So, I'd like to ask you to wait at least 15 minutes before eating or drinking anything.

    To heal emotional-eating tendencies, we must develop an inner-directed habit of listening to the still, small voice within us. Instead of pouring food into our gut in order to silence it, we must listen to what our gut is trying to tell us.

+ ***Analyze your food craving.*** During that 15-minute waiting period, analyze the source of your emotional discomfort by working backwards. You can use the chart in the back of this book, you could read the chapter corresponding to your food craving, or you could analyze the components yourself.

First start with the texture of the food:

— *If it is crunchy*, your core feelings are either Anger or Tension. Variations on these two feelings include resentment, feeling betrayed, feeling overwhelmed, feeling used, bitterness, and irritability.

— *If it is soft or creamy*, then your core feelings are either Fear or Shame. Variations on these feelings include anxiety, embarrassment, insecurity, the impostor syndrome, feeling unworthy, and guilt.

— *If it is chewy*, then your core feeling is a combination of either Fear or Shame mixed with either Anger or Tension. Variations on these combination feelings include jealousy (Fear with Anger); confusion (Tension with Shame); dread that something awful is about to happen (Fear with Tension); and self-loathing (Anger with Shame).

Foods often have a combination of textures; for example, rocky road ice cream has all three textures. The ice cream is creamy, the nuts are crunchy, and the marshmallows are chewy. With these texture combinations, look at the predominant one first. That's your most pressing emotion. Then look at the second most-noticeable texture, then the third. This process will serve as a mirror for you, so you can see which emotion is troubling you to the greatest degree.

Don't worry about being right or wrong in deciding which texture is most predominant or noticeable. *You* are the only person who can decide that a particular texture in a food stands out the most. For example, one person with rocky road ice cream cravings might say that the crunchy nuts are the most noticeable textures. That's because his or her emotional issues are different than yours. That person is more troubled by Anger or Tension than any other type of feeling.

If this is confusing, please keep reading. The methods I use for food-craving analysis are actually pretty straightforward and simple. As you read on, my methods will become clearer to you. Still, if you prefer, you can use the chart at the back of the book instead of performing self-analyses.

✦ *Next, look at the type of food you are craving.* Each chapter lists the reasons for the different types of foods commonly craved. Are you craving nuts, spicy food, cheese, chocolate, noodles? Every food type signifies a different underlying emotion. If you are craving a combination of foods, as in our rocky road ice cream example, then you'll be combining the emotional meaning of vanilla ice cream, nuts, and chewy caramel and marshmallow cravings: You are feeling angry because of your too-tight schedule and heavy responsibilities (nut cravings); you just want to relax (ice cream cravings) and have fun (nut cravings), but are afraid that would create more problems (caramel and marshmallow cravings).

✦ *Ask yourself, "Am I willing to face this issue right now?"* Stand or sit silently, so you can better hear the answer. Instantly, your appetite will tell you something like, "Of course!" or "Yes," or "I'm afraid to admit it, but I am upset." As soon as you've admitted your feelings to yourself, you'll feel a deliciously warm sense of relief (which feels even better than eating!). You'll feel lighter, less frustrated. And you'll be *so* happy to be free of out-of-control food cravings.

The freedom I experience when I analyze my own food cravings and then feel the cravings vanish is similar to leaving a really noisy environment and transporting myself to a peaceful and quiet place. It's such a relief!

✦ *Take action, NOW!* What is one action you can take today that will help ease your burden? Problems don't go away on their own; often they get worse. Instead of procrastinating and carrying the burden of this problem, think of one way to move toward relief. If no answers are apparent, meditate, pray, or otherwise quiet all the noise in your mind and body. Then affirm: *"All the wisdom of the universe is within me right this very moment. I trust that my Divine plan is in order and working right now. I release all fear and doubt, and listen to my inner guide."*

✦ ***Look for the "butterfly feeling" of love.*** As discussed in Chapter 3, the butterfly feeling is that little flutter of love, excitement, and good feelings that always resides in your gut. It's similar to the feeling of childlike excitement on a holiday or a birthday. Find that feeling and ask it to expand and envelop you in feelings of free-spirited enjoyment. You can ride that feeling upward to a higher consciousness and elevated emotion just as a kite rides a gust of wind toward the sun. This seemingly simple exercise will make you feel like you've fallen deeply in love with the most wonderful person. And, as a result, your appetite will dissipate. (Once you try this exercise, you'll know what I mean.)

By relaxing and enveloping yourself in love, your gut has no room to harbor Fear, or its manifestations of Anger, Tension, or Shame. A negative and a positive emotion cannot simultaneously exist. In this quiet and calm state of love, you can hear your gut feelings. Soon, you will know what you need to do to rectify your situation. Continue to release your fears and do what you must to bring your life back into spiritual order and harmony.

ॐ   ॐ   ॐ

SOUL FOOD: HEALING THE ROOT OF CONSTANT CRAVINGS

A s I've mentioned before, and I will reiterate again: excessive food cravings are a signal that something in our life is troubling us. The purest part of ourselves, which I call the "soul," is very honest and always acknowledges when something's amiss. That pure and unadulterated part of you is always speaking to you, guiding you, and helping you. When we get too busy or doubtful to listen to our soul, it has no choice but to deliver louder messages with cravings, pain, or insomnia. Our true self, deep down, wants us to wake up and pay attention.

The methods detailed in this chapter will reduce your cravings to the point where you'll regain your freedom of choice and composure. Instead of feeling like you *need* chocolate, you'll feel free to choose whether to eat it or not. Your cravings won't be controlling you; *you'll* be in charge of what you put into your mouth.

If you have the same cravings on a consistent basis, there are some underlying factors to examine. In essence, a Constant Craving is like a record with a scratch in it. The song skips, playing the same three notes over and over and over. Well, your Constant Craving is like the repetitious skipping of those same three notes.

Ninety-nine percent of the time, the "cure" for a Constant Craving involves making some change in your life—changing your relationship or communication habits, changing your work habits, changing your exercise habits, changing your sleeping habits.

There's no question that change can be difficult and frightening! It requires a lot of thought, patience, and practice. Sometimes it involves discussions with other people, where we have to admit our vulnerable thoughts or emotions to someone else. Change triggers fears that we will lose love. No wonder we prefer to avoid even acknowledging the situation to ourselves!

The truth is that when we act in love, more love comes into our lives. It's the law of sowing and reaping: we receive what we freely give. When we replace fear with love, we attract only positive situations and people into our lives. Remember the last time you were deeply in love? Didn't the world seem extra-beautiful? Didn't people tell you that you were glowing? When you are in love, you are irresistible on many levels.

By "in love," though, I don't necessarily mean a love relationship. I mean living in a state of love. You'll live in love by expanding on the "butterfly feeling" and through consistent spiritual work, such as meditation, prayer, and affirmations.

A Constant Craving is a signal that some situation needs to be corrected. Our soul is banging on our stomach like a person desperately trying to get our attention. The soul is screaming at us, "You've got to do something!" But we're terrified of taking the chance that things will actually become worse if we make changes. Constant Cravings, then, are internal wars between our fears and our soul.

Soul Food

When we're emotionally hungry (as described in Chapters 2 and 3), the desire for food feels like we're starving. Even though you just ate a full meal, a sudden attack of emotional hunger will have you believing that your stomach is completely empty. You feel hungry!

As you've been reading and as I've said quite a few times in this book, your stomach isn't hungry. It's your heart and your soul that are feeling hungry, deprived, or empty.

Each type of Constant Craving signals different unfulfilled needs, including needs for fun, affection, appreciation, romance, and relaxation. When these needs aren't met, Fear, or its manifestations of Anger, Tension, or Shame, are always involved:

— *Fear* keeps us from making changes that could improve our life. These include fears of failure, fears of abandonment, fears of rejection, and fears of being unworthy or being seen as an impostor.

— *Anger* stems from our unmet needs. This is especially true when we blame our circumstances on some outside force that is preventing us from improving our life. Some people blame their spouse, children, their upbringing, lack of education, their sex, their race, or their finances. This blame is rooted in the fear of taking responsibility for making changes. It is much easier to blame outside forces for thwarting our goals.

— *Tension* is the physical and emotional manifestation of life stress. Everyone experiences stress, yet we experience more life stress whenever we move away from our life's work and Divine path. As long as we work in harmony with our purpose, the universe helps us along. We feel strong, energized, and renewed.

— *Shame* means feeling unworthy, insecure, unqualified, or inadequate. It means doubting your abilities or goodness. Sometimes, Shame stems from guilt about real or imagined misdeeds. The only misdeed worth putting energy into is this: assessing whether or not you are listening to the inner voice that guides you. When we walk away from what we know is right, our self-esteem suffers. Shame is the result.

The common thread throughout every Constant Craving, though, is a need for "Soul Food."

Now, I'm not referring to Southern fried food, but self-loving thoughts and gestures you perform for yourself, for your soul—the actions that make you feel as if you're radiating good feelings.

Here are a few ways to feed yourself Soul Food:

✦ ***Seek spiritual stimulation.*** Remember when you were younger, how you'd have those deep conversations about the meaning of life? Didn't that feel good? That was a form of Soul Food that—if you're like most busy people—you haven't experienced in some time.

Busy adults have to *plan* ways to receive spiritual stimulation. Like most goals, it won't happen by accident. Here are some suggestions for progressing on your spiritual path:

— *Have a heart-to-heart conversation* with your spouse, best friend, or roommate. It will bring you both closer, and emotional intimacy is a form of Soul Food.

— *Join a spiritual study group.* Many community newspapers feature announcements about groups that study and discuss *A Course in Miracles*, the Bible, or great philosophical writings. Take your pick! Anything that stimulates your soul and opens your heart with love and childlike awe is a form of Soul Food.

— *Read or listen to material of a spiritual nature.* I'd like to suggest any of Marianne Williamson's books or taped lectures (available through my publisher, Hay House, Inc.). I am particularly fond of her books, *A Return to Love* and *Illuminata,* which are truly great spiritual/metaphysical works with a lot of practical advice interspersed throughout. Just as our bodies always change in response to regular exercise, so too does our outlook change in response to regular prayer and meditation, according to Marianne Williamson. She points out that, even if we're not enjoying the physical exercise as we perform it, our body still benefits. Prayer and meditation are the same, and "cannot not work," she told me. "When you pray, you receive peace of mind."[1]

— *Develop a creative hobby.* These are physical outlets for your soul's creative expressions. If you're a naturally creative person who hasn't been artistic lately, you'll love the natural high you'll feel when you reconnect with this part of yourself! If creative ventures are unnatural to you, there are dozens of community college courses. Find one that interests you, and sign up today! Some creative hobbies to try: painting, photography, sculpture, stained glasswork, sewing, crafts, jewelry making, playing a musical instrument, dancing, writing, film-making, calligraphy, and quilting.

✦ *Create an "Alone Oasis."* Do you have a little room or cubbyhole that belongs to only you? If not, I'd like to suggest that you create one. If you live with other people, you need an Alone Oasis—a space where you can quietly sit and think, write, or read. Every home, no matter how small, has some little corner where you could put a desk and comfortable chair (readily available at any secondhand furniture store for a reasonable cost). Think of this as an investment in yourself! Decorate your corner or room with reflections of your soul. That means decorating only with the photos, plants, knick-knacks, stuffed animals, or paintings that really make you happy.

✦ *Give yourself a daily time-out.* We all need a breather, a timeout when we can meditate and just be alone with our thoughts and our feelings. All day long, you're pummeled by the noise and energies of so many people—your boss, your kids, the clerks, the customers, the dog! Now you need to take the equivalent of a shower, by cleansing your soul of all that noise. During your time-out, be careful not to try to block out thoughts or feelings with food or other distractions. Just get away by yourself for at least five minutes. If alone time is difficult to attain, go sit in your car, take a walk to the mailbox, or sit in the bathroom.

+ *Go on a Negativity Diet.* Those of us who are highly sensitive absorb negativity from our surroundings. Even though you are a very strong person who is smart and aware, outside negative influences can still invade your heart, mind, and soul. Just as some physical diseases are considered contagious, so is the mental illness of negative, unhealthy thinking. If you surround yourself with negative people and influences long enough, you will start to see the world as they see it. You will adopt their unhealthy "ain't life awful" viewpoints, and you will find that it becomes second nature to you, too.

You can really tell how much negativity you've been absorbing by going on a Negativity Diet. The first time I did this, I couldn't believe the results! I felt so light and happy, and life seemed to reward me with small miracles. I recommend that you try it for one week, and see if you don't feel many pounds lighter. This is one of the most powerful therapeutic tools I've ever used. Every one of my clients who has gone on the Negativity Diet has reported great results: improved relationships, increased self-confidence, and fewer worries and fears. As with any diet, you can tailor it to fit your lifestyle and goals. An ultra-low Negativity Diet will produce the fastest results, but it also requires the most determination to stick with. A moderate Negativity Diet is not as stringent, but the results are not as powerful. Here's how to go on a Negativity Diet:

— *Eliminate all contact with negative media.* Avoid any television or radio program, magazine or newspaper story, or any movie that has an "ain't life awful" theme, or that is reporting the latest crisis, disease, or consumer scam. If there's anything really important that you need to know, someone will alert you.

Later, if you "add back" negative media stories into your diet, guard your thinking. We can choose to be objective and not swallow journalism hype as the ultimate truth. Yes, hysteria sells newspapers and the 11:00 news. But does it help your soul find comfort?

— *As I touched on above, avoid negative, critical, or judgmental people.* Their spiritual sickness can be contagious! Refer these folks to a professional helper if you feel they need a shoulder to cry on. Avoid their company and telephone calls for one week (if not permanently) because your soul needs some time away from their negative influences. You'll be amazed at the difference this step will make in increasing your energy level!

Many of my clients tell me, "But my spouse is negative! How can I avoid negativity when I live with a negative person?" I always remind them that a negative relationship is a two-way agreement. If you are living with a negative mate, know that he or she is responding in part to your behavior. Right or wrong, most spouses tend to take your happiness or unhappiness personally. As I wrote in my book, *In the Mood,* if you are happy, your significant other will feel great. If you are unhappy, he or she feels wounded. When you shine with happiness from your Negativity Diet, your mate will be drawn to you and feel validated and relieved when he or she sees you expressing contentment.

The bottom line is that you have the power to heal much of the negativity in your relationships. At the same time, I wouldn't want you to blame yourself for any abusiveness or hostility in your mate. Perhaps at one time, your self-esteem was somewhat low, and you attracted a mate that validated a lack of self-worth. As you grow stronger, your relationships will definitely change. The ones worth saving will heal. The others will naturally fade away. And you will be fine in accepting all these changes, knowing that you are safe, strong, and loved.

— *Avoid thinking negative thoughts or speaking negative words*. Our thoughts are magnets and messengers. Guard your thinking, and only send out messages of love, optimism, and success. In this way, you attract those very qualities into your life. For one week, avoid complaining, criticizing, judging, or "awfulizing" about anyone or anything (even gossip about movie stars!). Your soul will breathe a sigh of relief, as it no longer has to repel negative influences with Constant Cravings.

✦ *Use affirmations.* This is the main course of the Soul Food menu. Affirmations are *the* definitive tool for overcoming the Fear of Change. Our fears usually stem from: a lack of self-confidence; a lack of belief in our talents, intelligence or abilities; a belief that we don't deserve better; fears that if we "rock the boat" or complain, others will abandon, fire, or divorce us; fears that we are impostors not deserving success; fears that things will get worse and that we won't be able to return to our present safety levels; and fears that our goals are impossible and unattainable.

After a while, you begin to believe these fears, but the fears actually stem from a distrust of our gut feelings that tell us to make changes in our lives. We doubt that we have enough time, creativity, intelligence, or money to heed our gut feelings.

Affirmations Can Heal Your Life

Affirmations will help you remember the truth about you: that God would never give you an assignment without also backing it up with talent. God is perfect, whole, and complete and you were made in His image and likeness. When you go for your gut-feeling goals, there is always a higher purpose that will benefit other people.

Lately, affirmations have gotten a bad rap by some of the media who have derided them as being naive and an outgrowth of the 12-Step movement. Well, I used affirmations to radically transform my life, many years ago. If it hadn't been for affirmations, I'd still be a narrow-minded and fearful woman, a fat, unhappy, uneducated housewife who was very depressed because I knew I wasn't living the life I was meant to live. I remember feeling like a car stuck in the mud, with wheels spinning full speed but going nowhere. So I ate food to mask my distress. Yet, with my metaphysical upbringing (I'm a third-generation metaphysician), I'd learned the incredible power of visualizations and affirmations. I visualized my dream of being a bestselling author and psychologist, and since I was too poor back then to purchase a prerecorded affirmation tape, I made my own. On the tape, I dictated many self-loving concepts and included plenty of positive thoughts about my career and weight.

Some of my affirmations included, "I am a bestselling author," "I appear on national talk shows," and "My figure is very attractive." Believe me—at the time, those affirmations seemed like lines out of a science fiction film; they were so far from the reality of my life! Yet, they were my deep-down truths. Those affirmations represented the life I was supposed to have.

I listened to that tape day and night. It was my soul's food, and I was so, so hungry for the loving thoughts that the tape provided! At first, the positive words sounded foreign, and I didn't care for the sound of my own voice. That was a sign of how low my self-esteem was! After a couple of weeks of daily listening, I started "hearing" the positive messages in my mind without the tape even being on. I would be at the store, and my mind would replay these positive messages about me being a likeable person who attracted loving friends.

The positive messages became ingrained in my thinking, and I developed a healthy love relationship with myself. I had no need to binge-eat on ice cream, since I was no longer depressed. I stopped eating crispy English muffins swimming in butter, since I no longer felt as stressed.

I hope you will choose to increase your self-love and self-confidence with the use of an affirmation tape. At the end of each of the following chapters, I've included affirmations that correspond to each particular food craving. In the food craving chart in the final chapter, you'll find dozens of affirmations geared toward healing your appetite.

When we feel overwhelming hunger for a food, the underlying emotions are Fear, Anger, Tension, and Shame. Fighting the emotions is useless; they only become stronger and try to fight you back. Don't waste one precious moment attempting to battle or ignore these emotions!

The only solution is to affirm "replacement" emotions. Invite positive emotional houseguests into your heart, and the negative houseguests will scurry. Once again, here is that wonderful affirmation for inviting love and light into your soul's house:

I Forgive, Accept, and Trust my Self.

This is your replacement FATS acronym. It's an instant appetite reducer, as well!

I like to think of affirmations as a way to increase your "Mental Metabolism." They are, in effect, appetite-suppressing thoughts.

𝖾𝐚 𝖾𝐚 𝖾𝐚

THE SCIENCE OF
FOOD CRAVINGS

CHOCOLATE CRAVINGS: HUNGRY FOR LOVE

Every year, Americans spend five billion dollars a year on chocolate. Ironically, that is roughly how much money is spent on weight-loss methods. Clearly, we are a nation of chocoholics. But, for thousands of people (especially women), chocolate cravings are no joke. They are a serious problem, affecting weight and self-esteem.

You may have heard that chocolate contains the same chemical that the brain creates when we're feeling romantic love. This chemical, *phenylethylamine* (pronounced fennel-ethyl-a-meen) and abbreviated as PEA, has the same properties whether found in chocolate or in the brain.

PEA is so powerfully mood-altering that it used to be a prescribed medication! Until the early 1980s, PEA was the main ingredient in a pill called MDMA. Then it was declared an illegal drug and was taken off the market. Today, the same pill is sold on the streets as "Ecstasy" or "X."

MDMA triggers feelings of euphoria. It's been said that you could put two mortal enemies in the same room, give them MDMA, and they'd be arm-in-arm best buddies within one hour. Marriage counselors used to give MDMA to couples to ease their tension and hostility. The pill made couples feel warm and fuzzy toward one another, and they'd soon kiss and make up.

Today, Ecstasy is a popular black-market drug. Since it is a form of metha-amphetamine, those who take Ecstasy are risking serious cardiovascular problems. Currently, researchers at the University of California at Davis are studying MDMA to look for possible beneficial or therapeutic uses for the drug.

With MDMA as an ingredient, it's no wonder chocolate cravings are so pervasive!

Chocolate: Queen of Cravings

In my surveys of clients and audience members, chocolate is always the number-one food that is craved. "If only I could quit craving chocolate, I could lose some weight," is a phrase I hear constantly. Other researchers have also concluded that chocolate is the number-one food craving, especially among women.[1]

Why do we crave chocolate to such a degree? Why do women, in particular, struggle with chocolate cravings? There are five possible reasons:

1. Love and emotional attachments are so important to women, and chocolate creates the feeling of being loved, cherished, and understood.

2. Our hormonal shifts throughout our menstrual cycle trigger cravings (see Chapter 8).

3. More women than men seek help for depression, and chocolate is an excellent, albeit temporary, antidepressant.

4. Women who do too much, who attempt Superwoman lifestyles, sometimes use chocolate to boost their energy.

Women Who Crave Love

In 1993, I gave a written survey to 150 females to determine their opinions on which elements of life lead to the greatest happiness. These were members of social organizations, such as Soroptomist or the American Association of University Women, who agreed to help me with my research. Those surveyed were not currently in therapy, and all of them defined themselves as "happy with their lives." Most were college graduates employed in careers such as teaching, management, or business ownership.

I asked the women to list the "most important" and "second most important" factors responsible for their current satisfaction. Under "most important," the majority listed "High self-esteem" as the most important ingredient in happiness. The second most frequently answered item—and this surprised me—was a "good spouse or lover." "Children" was the third most frequently chosen response.

When I combined the total responses for what these women named as the most, and second most, important factors leading to happiness, "good spouse or lover" ended up being the top answer!

I also asked the women two other questions that yielded interesting results:

1. What is the biggest factor influencing your happiness or unhappiness with your life right now?

2. What, if anything, do you feel is missing from your life at present?

What do you think were the top answers for these two questions? You've probably guessed it: these women—all with successful careers—rated relationships, love, and marriage as the most important influences on their happiness or unhappiness, *above all other factors!*

Of course, many men crave emotional intimacy, romance, and love, too. Some studies show that, today, more men than ever before are expressing desires for commitment and marriage. And, guess what? Those men are often chocoholics.

You see, chocoholism is a cry for love, intimacy, and romance. It is the perfect antidepressant for the lovesick. Just look at the melting pot of feel-good properties in chocolate:

— The high-fat content soothes feelings of emptiness, insecurity, or loneliness.
— Its high-carbohydrate content triggers production of the brain's feel-good chemical, serotonin.
— It also contains a serotonin-like substance called *diphenylamine,* which appears to promote feelings of calm and serenity.
— The stimulants in chocolate—PEA, theobromine, tyramine, and caffeine—are instant pick-me-ups.
— Chocolate's appeal may be due, in part, to having a flavor that equally combines sweet, salty, bitter, and sour tastes in a perfect balance.
— Pyrazine, a chemical that is found in the odor of chocolate, triggers the pleasure center in the brain.[2]
— The texture can be creamy if you need comfort, or crunchy if you're angry over your love life.

Sometimes when I discuss this craving for love, people get defensive and insist, "It isn't true!" It's difficult to admit when our love life is unfulfilling, because along with that admission comes an acknowledgment that we must make changes. We all naturally resist change, fearing that things will get even worse than they already are. Instead of making changes, we medicate our love misery with chocolate. Cynthia is an example:

A member of the studio audience at a television talk show where I was discussing food cravings, Cynthia stood up and said she was constantly craving chocolate. "What causes this, and how can I control it?" she wanted to know.

Cynthia had provided me with the customary starting point in food-craving analysis—pointing out the object of her craving—chocolate. Chocolate cravings almost always signal unmet needs for love. But since unmet love needs take many different forms, I asked Cynthia about the second factor—texture—to find out more.

"What type of chocolate do you crave?" I asked her.

Cynthia explained that she usually binged on crunchy, crispy chocolate bars. Crunchy textures often signal frustration or anger in the love area, so I asked Cynthia the next logical question.

"How's your love life?"

"Fine," she replied, with a deadpan expression. I noticed that her mouth twitched as she said the word.

Bingo! Cynthia's cravings were a creation of her own denial. When she told me her love life was fine, I knew I had zeroed in on the right issue. I've never met a chocolate craver yet who was completely happy with his or her love life.

"Constant cravings for crunchy chocolate usually mean frustration or anger with your love life," I told her. "Does this fit your situation?" All the while, the cameras were filming this conversation, and the signals were being beamed out live. I had stuck out my neck once again, because I truly believed in my food-craving analysis research.

"Well..." Cynthia looked down. Then she blurted out her story. She was newly married to a military man who had been sent out to sea two weeks after their marriage. Cynthia was extremely angry about the situation, yet she felt that admitting these feelings to herself was a futile gesture. At this time, however, she seemed visibly relieved to discuss her feelings, and she sat down with a smile.

As I've mentioned, chocolate is predominantly a "woman's craving." Yet, I have also worked with many men who have struggled with overwhelming desires for chocolate. Men, just like women who crave chocolate, are the romantics of the world. Chocoholics are usually those who wish that life could be one long romance novel. We often have unrealistic expectations about relationships, expecting red roses, love songs, and poetry. When these expectations are dashed, we often feel let down.

Some chocoholic romantics are unhappy with their love lives because they consistently choose inappropriate or incompatible mates. Some, like my client Ted, are romantically dissatisfied because Fear and Shame keep them from seeking a love partner in the first place.

A 28-year-old middle manager at a top manufacturing company, Ted is hard-working, smart, and friendly. Except when he gets around women—then he clams up. "I feel so afraid whenever I'm near an attractive woman," he admitted to me.

Instead of pursuing the relationship he desires, Ted throws himself into his work. He's 50 pounds overweight, something he attributes to his constant cravings for Reese's peanut butter cups. "If I could just stop eating that candy, I know I could lose weight," Ted complained. He had tried conventional diets, but had always regained his weight when his cravings for peanut butter and chocolate resurfaced.

Ted's chocolate and peanut butter cravings signify a yearning for love and fun, respectively. Basically, Ted worked all day and went straight home every night. He had shut the door on love and fun and had to make some life changes if he was ever going to fulfill either need. This meant signing up for interesting classes and sports activities where he would have the opportunity to meet new friends and maybe bump into the woman of his dreams. With his needs for love and fun being fulfilled, Ted could let go of his Reese's cravings.

The chocolate/love connection was studied by Margorie Schuman, a professor at the California School of Professional Psychology. Schuman found that people who use chocolate to medicate or cover up depression, tension, or irritability tend to exhibit certain personality traits:

+ They are dramatic, flamboyant and have a great need to be the center of attention.
+ They have frequent mood swings.
+ They tend to fall in love more easily than others.
+ They becomes devastated by romantic rejection.
+ They are ultra-sensitive to the approval or disapproval of others.[3]

Addicted to Love?

In her book, *A Natural History of Love,* Diane Ackerman discusses how being hooked on the natural high of PEA (the brain chemical also found in chocolate) can lead to relationship problems:

> When two people find one another attractive, their bodies quiver with a gush of PEA, a molecule that speeds up the flow of information between nerve cells. An amphetaminelike chemical, PEA whips the brain into a frenzy of excitement, which is why lovers feel euphoric, rejuvenated, optimistic and energized, happy to sit up talking all night or making love for hours on end. Because amphetamine, or "speed," is addictive—even the body's naturally made speed—some people become what Michael Liebowitz and Donald Klein of the New York

State Psychiatric Institute refer to as "attraction junkies," needing a romantic relationship to feel excited by life.

Driven by a chemical hunger, they choose unsuitable partners. Soon the relationship crumbles, or they find themselves rejected. In either case, tortured by lovesick despair, they plummet into a savage depression, which they try to cure by falling in love again. Liebowitz and Klein think this roller-coaster is fueled by a craving for PEA. When they gave some attraction junkies MAO inhibitors—antidepressants that can subdue PEA and other neurotransmitters—the researchers were amazed to find how quickly their patients improved. No longer craving PEA, they were able to choose partners more calmly and realistically. All this strongly suggests that when we fall in love, the brain drenches itself in PEA, a chemical that makes us feel pleasure, rampant excitement, and well-being. A sweet fix, love.[4]

When we're in love, we quite often lose our appetite, feeling that our emotions are taking precedence over all other mundane problems. Author/lecturer Marianne Williamson calls this feeling a state of "positive denial," when we are recognizing the truth of perfection in our self and our partner.[5]

We crave chocolate because we yearn for those free-spirited feelings of love. My client, LeAnne, recognized that she ate less whenever she was in love:

When LeAnne didn't have a boyfriend, she'd bake and eat brownies every day. Her chocolate cravings hinged upon whether or not she had a love relationship going!

LeAnne's weight swung up and down by 20 pounds, contingent upon the state of her love life. Her method of dieting was to try and control the chocolate cravings by staying in love. Here is how she did it: LeAnne would dress in very flattering and somewhat revealing clothes. She'd go to a nightclub and flirt with an attractive man. LeAnne was not looking for a steady relationship; instead, her goal was to find a man who would act as her love object. It didn't matter what the man acted like, looked like, or what type of job he had. What mattered was whether or not he triggered romantic chemistry in her, so she could quit craving chocolate.

Her life was chaotic when she first came in for therapy. She had so many men calling her, and yet LeAnne was not "in love" in the way she truly craved. She was using these men as a way of sticking to her diet, and her temporary infatuations were poor substitutes for the love she desired.

In therapy, LeAnne discovered that infatuations are like junk food, while love represents genuine nourishment. LeAnne learned how to increase the amount of love she felt for herself and her life, and was able to release her chocolate cravings naturally.

Emergency Solutions for Chocolate Cravings

Chocolate cravings, which are based on unfulfilled desires for love, turn into physically based cravings when we treat ourselves in unloving ways. Our serotonin and energy levels are drained by stress-filled days, too-tight schedules, unhealthful eating, and lack of exercise. We then turn to chocolate to feel better.

Chocolate cravings can be temporarily masked by drinking beverages that contain some of the same stimulating properties as chocolate:

— *Ginger ale*. Its high tyramine content can relieve chocolate cravings.
— *Pekoe tea*. High in chocolate's other stimulating ingredient, theobromine, tea is simultaneously soothing and stimulating.
— *Soy milk*. Contains huge amounts of tyramine, as well as many vitamins and minerals.

— *Diet soda.* There is some evidence that phenylalanine, one of the amino acids in aspartame (NutraSweet), stimulates brain production of phenylethylamine, the same "love drug" found in chocolate.[6] I don't recommend drinking a lot of diet soda, but one 12-ounce can per day may temporarily curtail your cravings.

— *Coffee.* The mere smell of coffee can alleviate chocolate cravings. When you open the can or brew a pot, it's a delightful sensory experience because a chemical called *pyrozine* is entering your brain via your nose. (Have you ever noticed that coffee smells better than it tastes? This is why!) Pyrozine triggers the pleasure center of your brain, and its odor can be found in all the members of the nut family, including coffee and chocolate.[7]

Here are some other emergency solutions for out-of-control chocolate cravings:

✦ ***Eat nonfat chocolate.*** Some people combat chocolate cravings by eating nonfat chocolate frozen yogurt or fat-free brownies or chocolate cookies. You probably already know that fat-free doesn't necessarily mean low-calorie. Yogurt is probably the best choice of the fat-free chocolate choices in terms of calories, and many women swear that chocolate yogurt combats premenstrual chocolate cravings.

✦ ***Exercise.*** Aerobic-type exercise will boost serotonin levels, improve your mood, help relieve premenstrual cramps, and suppress your appetite in general. Exercise also increases the metabolic rate, meaning that you'll burn calories more efficiently throughout the day. This rise in metabolism can last as long as 12 hours after a workout.[8]

Healing Chocolate Cravings

As my client Ted discovered, the only lasting cure for chocolate cravings comes from the inside out. This means fulfilling your need for love by treating yourself like you were the most special person in the world (which you are!). It means teaching your partner what you will and won't accept in a relationship. It also means refusing to settle for a relationship that is abusive in any way.

Stay in love with your life by expanding the "butterfly feelings" in your stomach. Any time you start to feel unloved, go into a quiet space and completely focus on your gut. Look for the slightest inkling of a butterfly in your stomach; the feeling that you're just about to open a wonderful present or like you've just won the lottery. Consciously expand that feeling, as if you are riding the butterfly feeling up into the air. Soon, your heart will feel soft and warm. You will experience identical feelings to being newly in love. These are the ones you are trying to reproduce by eating chocolate.

With practice, you will be able to remain in a state of romantic love all day, every day. By living in this state of love, you will be able to suppress your appetite; and your face, actions, and words will glow with happiness. You will also naturally attract loving people into your life.

Above all, say these affirmations to yourself over and over. You'll get the most benefit by repeating them twice a day, every day, for one month:

Affirmations for Chocolate Cravings

&⬥ I deserve love.

&⬥ I am love, and love shines through me.

&⬥ I am full of love, through and through.

&⬥ I am experiencing a state of bliss throughout my body.

&⬥ I am lovable and loved, right this very moment.

&⬥ I attract loving people into my life.

&⬥ My friends are loving, giving, and considerate.

&⬥ I deserve love just for being who I am.

&⬥ I ask for what I need in my relationships.

&⬥ I ask for, receive, and listen to, Divine guidance, with respect to my relationships.

In the next chapter, we'll look at the different forms of chocoholism with the help of a quiz that will pinpoint the intensity of your chocolate cravings. By understanding why and how your cravings occur, you'll be better equipped to overcome them.

&⬥   &⬥   &⬥

ARE YOU A CHOCOHOLIC?
(A Quiz)

Have you ever said to yourself, "I could lose weight if it wasn't for all the chocolate candy and ice cream I eat"? Do you consider yourself a chocoholic?

For a long time, chocoholics have been the subject of bad jokes and have even been regarded with suspicion. "That's just an excuse to eat a lot of candy bars," non-chocoholics sometimes contend. "Just use your will power and eat only *one* chocolate," we're told over and over again.

Easy for *them* to say—that's like telling an alcoholic to drink just one beer! For many chocoholics, there's no such thing as *one* chocolate butter cream, or *one* milk chocolate candy bar, or *one* piece of chocolate cake. Most people know whether they're chocoholics or not. But just in case you're not quite sure, or if you don't know to what degree or what type of chocoholic you are, please take this quiz:

ARE YOU A CHOCOHOLIC?

True or False:

1. I frequently crave chocolate.
2. My favorite food has chocolate in it.
3. At times, I go on chocolate binges and eat an entire carton of chocolate ice cream, a bag of chocolate cookies, most of a chocolate cake, or a large amount of chocolate candy.

4. *For women only:* I crave chocolate right before my menstrual cycle.
5. It seems that I always eat more chocolate in the winter, and I gain weight during the cold months as a result.
6. I have gone to great lengths to seek out my favorite chocolate treat (e.g., driven several miles out of my way, spent money I couldn't afford, etc.).
7. I usually eat chocolate treats when others aren't around, and I even hide the empty candy wrappers so that others won't know what I've eaten.
8. After I eat chocolate, I feel guilty, and am angry at myself.
9. Just the sight or smell of chocolate is enough to make me desire it.
10. I think I'm a hopeless romantic; I fall in love easily, and I can't get enough of romantic movies or books.
11. The best thing about chocolate is its delicious taste.
12. If I were stranded on a deserted isle, I'd definitely want chocolate to be one of the supplies in my survival pack.
13. Life without chocolate wouldn't be much fun.
14. The last time I broke up with a lover, I was depressed for days, and I ate more chocolate as a result.
15. It really seems like I crave chocolate most during the holidays.
16. Every time I take a bite of chocolate, I lose total control of my appetite and I want to eat every bit of chocolate I can get my hands on.
17. I've noticed that I feel really good when I'm eating chocolate. It's like a natural high.
18. Others have kidded me or commented that I seem to like chocolate more than "normal" people do.
19. Sometimes I use chocolate as a pick-me-up when I'm feeling tired or depressed.
20. I have fond childhood memories surrounding the eating of chocolate.

21. Speaking of childhood, as a kid I used to hide when I ate chocolate. I never let my parents or siblings know when I was eating chocolate treats.

22. It seems that I'm able to keep the weight off until the fall holidays from Halloween until New Year's Day. There's just so much chocolate being passed around during those times of the year that I always gain weight.

23. To me, the more chocolate flavor, the better. I'll always opt for "double fudge" chocolate ice cream instead of light milk chocolate or (yuch!) plain vanilla.

24. I usually think of chocolate as being a "bad" food—bad for my weight, bad for my health—but so delicious that I allow myself to be "naughty" and eat some.

25. I can't stand the taste of carob. To me, it's fake chocolate.

26. When my mom used to ask me what flavor cake I'd like for my birthday, I'd *always* ask for chocolate cake with chocolate frosting.

27. I like chocolate more than anyone else in my family does.

28. I go on chocolate "kicks"; that is, I'll like a certain type of chocolate and eat only that type until I get sick of it. Then I'll choose a different type of chocolate until I get sick of that kind.

29. I only seem to binge on chocolate when it contains refined sugar, such as a candy bar, cake, or ice cream. I don't feel like overeating when I have sugar-free chocolate candy, ice milk, or frozen yogurt.

30. After an argument with my mate, I usually crave or eat chocolate.

31. I feel happy and excited right before I'm about to eat my favorite chocolate treat.

32. If other people knew how much chocolate I really ate, I'd feel embarrassed—even humiliated.

33. To me, chocolate is a sensual food. I've noticed that chocolate's texture and taste arouse my sexual desires.

34. When I go to the movies, I'd rather eat chocolate candy than popcorn.
35. If my mate brought home my very favorite chocolate treat (ice cream, candy, cookies, etc.), I couldn't help but view it as an act of love.

How to Score Your Quiz:

Count the number of "true" answers you have, and then see which category below applies to you:

0 to 10:

You may enjoy an occasional chocolate, but you're not a chocoholic. You can take chocolate or leave it, and when ordering an ice cream cone or frozen yogurt, you often order vanilla or fruit flavors. When you eat sweets, it's frequently the hard-candy or pastry variety. In other words, chocolate is really no big deal to you. You may know or love a chocoholic, however; and to you, the whole subject of chocoholism is a mystery or a joke.

11 to 20:

You're a "borderline chocoholic" — that is, you like chocolate a lot, but your whole life doesn't revolve around it. Instead, you've probably noticed that chocolate is something you enjoy at regular intervals, perhaps if someone has happened to bring some in to work or to your home. You wouldn't turn it down if it were offered to you, but you wouldn't go out of your way to seek it out, either.

You've eaten your share of chocolate candy and cakes, and when dieting, you've sworn off all sweets and desserts. But as with others who are fond of chocolate, you've found that when it has been offered to you, it has meant the downfall of many of your weight-loss attempts.

21 to 29:

You are definitely a chocoholic and you know it. You prefer chocolate to any other flavor, and you wouldn't dream of ordering a vanilla ice cream cone. You've driven across town to get your favorite chocolate treat, even when you're short on time or money. You've eaten chocolate to celebrate good times, as well as to comfort yourself during the bad times.

During certain periods in your life, you've felt out of control around chocolate, like an alcoholic around alcohol, and there have been many times when you've felt you couldn't stop eating the chocolate candies or cookies in front of you. You know you're addicted to chocolate, at least psychologically, and you loathe diets because they make you give up your favorite food.

30 to 35:

You're the "ultimate chocoholic"—a hard-core addict who lives for the taste and smell of chocolate. You crave and eat chocolate every day, if not *several* times a day. You plan your day so that you'll have time to stop off at the market or the ice cream/frozen-yogurt shop to get your favorite chocolate treat.

Other people probably kid you about your chocolate obsession, but you don't care—at least not enough to ever stop eating it. In the past, you've sworn off chocolate, but you really think it's a losing battle and that you're a hopelessly incurable chocoholic.

What Type of Chocoholic Are You?

Now that you've analyzed the intensity of your chocoholism, it's important to determine what type of chocoholic you are. People tend to overeat chocolate in different ways and for a variety of reasons.

The first step involved in regaining control over your chocolate appetite is to find out what type of chocoholic you are, because any modifications in your eating habits need to correspond to your personality and behavior patterns. I can't emphasize this enough: Not all chocoholics are alike!

To discern your category, please review the answers you gave on the true/false questions and match them up to the descriptions below:

The Chocolate Lover. If you answered "true" to three or more of these questions: 10, 14, 30, 33, 35, then you are a Chocolate Lover. A Chocolate Lover is someone who has a strong need for romance and love. This person binges on the positive emotions produced by eating chocolate—feelings aroused by PEA—the same chemical your brain secretes during the early and romantic phases of love.

The Situational Chocoholic. If you answered "true" to three or more of these questions: 4, 5, 15, 22, 26, then you are a Situational Chocoholic. There are three general subcategories of Situational Chocoholics:

1. The woman who craves chocolate right before her menstrual cycle due to hormonal fluctuations.
2. The person who desires chocolate only during the cold winter months because of seasonally influenced depression.
3. The person who just craves chocolate when it happens to be around, especially during holidays.

The Chocolate Binger. If you answered "true" to three or more of these questions: 3, 6, 16, 28, 29, then you are a Chocolate Binger. This person literally cannot have one bite of chocolate without going all-out into an eating binge. Some Bingers only lose control with chocolate that contains certain ingredients, such as refined sugar or nuts. Other Bingers overeat certain *types* of chocolate treats, such as ice cream or cake.

The Euphoric Chocoholic. If you answered "true" to three or more of these questions: 9, 13, 17, 19, 31, then you are a Euphoric Chocoholic. The Euphoric Chocoholic experiences total and utter bliss when eating chocolate. This person usually describes eating chocolate as a "completely perfect experience," and the Euphoric Chocoholic would be hard-pressed to tell you which aspect of chocolate is more appealing: the taste, the smell, or the texture. All in all, the Euphoric Chocoholic derives a pronounced "high" from eating chocolate.

The Closet Chocoholic. If you answered "true" to three or more of these questions: 7, 8, 21, 24, 32, then you are a Closet Chocoholic. This person usually feels very guilty about eating anything labeled "fattening"—which includes chocolate. The Closet Chocoholic often hides while eating a favorite chocolate treat. He or she may also conceal candy bar wrappers in a purse or a car, or wait for family members to go to sleep so that the chocolate cake or ice cream can be eaten in blissful solitude.

Chocolate—A Love/Hate Relationship

Some chocoholics encompass a combination of more than one type. Others fall into every category of chocoholism. If you fit into one or more groups, you may find some comfort in knowing that you're not alone. Yet, you're probably also frustrated by the push-pull effect of chocolate in your life.

On the one hand, you don't want to live without chocolate. On the other hand, you feel that chocolate is the primary culprit behind your out-of-control eating.

As we discussed in the last chapter, though, the actual source of the problem is the desire for more love and excitement in your life.

Many recovering chocoholics find that as soon as they start practicing self-love, the moment they start to engage in more creative and inspiring activities, that's when they're able to begin releasing the hold that chocolate has on them!

DAIRY CRAVINGS:
THE ANTIDEPRESSANT FOODS

A s infants, we all craved and consumed a great deal of milk. Some researchers believe that our earliest cravings for milk are, in reality, cravings for the sweet lactose that is found in this dairy product.[1] Lactose is a form of sugar, and we have seen how all newborns prefer sweet tastes to any other. In fact, lactose intolerance almost never occurs before the age of one-and-a-half.[2]

But there are other properties of dairy products even more powerful than their inherently sweet taste. When you break down the ingredients of these milk-based products, you find an over-the-counter antidepressant—no prescription necessary!

Just look at the host of mood-altering properties in dairy products:

— *Tyramine,* a vasoactive substance highly abundant in cheese, acts as a stimulant.
— *Choline,* a primary ingredient in milk, has a soothing effect on the body.
— Another inherent property of milk is *L-tryptophan.* When dairy products are combined with carbohydrates (so competing amino acids don't interfere), L-tryptophan triggers the production of the brain chemical, serotonin. This creates a pleasant feel-good sensation. Common dairy-carbohydrate

combinations include ice cream, flavored yogurt, pizza, nachos with cheese, and pasta Alfredo.

In addition, the sugar in milk products boosts energy and mood, and the creamy smooth texture is comforting.

ANTI-DEPRESSANT EFFECTS OF DAIRY PRODUCTS

Ingredient/Characteristic	Effect on Mood/Energy
Choline	Soothing
L-tryptophan (when combined w/ carbs)	Calming
Sugar or lactose	Temporarily energizing
Creamy texture	Comforting

Common dairy product cravings are for ice cream, cheeses, sour cream, Alfredo sauces, and creamy salad dressings such as ranch, Roquefort, and blue cheese. Let's look at Rose's cravings, for example.

This 33-year-old marketing director and mother of two would binge-eat dairy products at salad bars. She'd rationalize that she was eating healthful, low-fat food. All the while, though, Rose's salads were composed of a small portion of lettuce, a few sprouts, mushrooms, and cherry tomatoes. The bulk of her salad consisted of shredded cheese, blue cheese crumbles, and ranch dressing — an antidepressant salad!

Since she was binge-eating dairy products in a crunchy form (from the vegetables), Rose's food-craving profile was that of someone who was both depressed and also frustrated or angry. Her dairy product choices were fairly high-fat ones, as well. This meant that she was probably struggling with some pangs of emptiness.

I asked Rose, "What is the irritating part of your life that is making you feel depressed right now?"

She looked at me, startled, with some of the color draining from her face. I had just blown her "cover"—the façade that told everyone that her life was perfect. Food-craving analysis does that! It goes straight to the heart of the emotions without beating around the bush.

Rose gulped, as if she were swallowing her pride while admitting that she was dealing with some perfectly natural emotions. "I guess I'm upset with my husband."

"What needs aren't being met right now?" I asked her.

"I would like to stay home with my children, but he says we can't afford it…" Her voice trailed off, and she turned her face away to dab at the tears streaming down her face.

Rose's heartbreak, her inability to realize her dream to be a full-time mother, had manifested in resentment toward her husband. Underneath her anger were these persistent protestations, "Dan should make more money and support all of us. A real man would know how important this is! He'd do *something* so I could be home where I belong, with our kids!"

Resentment and frustration, if ignored, eventually mutate into depression. This was the case with Rose. Instead of focusing on possible solutions, using goal-setting, affirmations, and rational discussions with her husband, Rose had chosen a different route. Her mental habit was to see herself as a victim and her husband as a jailkeeper. Yet, I had met her husband in their joint therapy sessions, and there was no evidence of abusiveness on his part. Rose had never mentioned any indication of mental or physical abuse, either.

Instead, Rose was afraid to confront the notion that her goals conflicted with the reality of her present life. She feared acknowledging the necessity for change if she was going to realize her dreams—either she'd have to cut down on living expenses, or figure out a way to make money from home.

I asked Rose to use quieting techniques (Chapter 7) so she could hear her gut feelings' direction. She was somewhat surprised by what came to her when she did so. She admitted to me at our next session that she intuited that she was supposed to open her own marketing company from home.

Healing her appetite, as well as starting and succeeding in a home-based business, required the same spiritual root: overcoming Fear and Anger. Here are the affirmations Rose used on her cassette tape to replace Fear and Anger with Forgiveness and Acceptance:

— I trust God's plans for me, and know that I am given talent along with a mission.
— When I walk the path that is right for me, all the details are taken care of.
— I can relax in God's arms, just as my children relax in my arms.
— Everything is perfect right now.
— When I concentrate on seeing excellent results, the in-between how's and why's take care of themselves.

Other Depression-Relieving Strategies

✦ **Get professional help, if necessary**. Depression can turn into the cancer of emotional illness if left untreated. It can be fatal, so it is not worth ignoring! If you've had any thoughts at all about suicide or wanting to disappear into nothingness, please put down this book right now and call the operator and ask for a suicide hotline number. Believe me, getting help will feel so good! It's a sign of strength to seek assistance, and you'll wonder why you waited so long. In the absence of suicidal thoughts, serious depression still requires professional intervention.

Please make an appointment with a doctor or therapist if you have experienced five or more of these symptoms on a continual basis for at least two weeks: depression; diminished interest or lack of pleasure in life; significant (over 5 percent of body weight) weight loss or gain; insomnia or hypersomnia (oversleeping); physical shaking or clumsiness; daily lack of energy; feelings of worthlessness or excessive guilt; difficulty in concentrating; recurrent thoughts about death or suicide. If you do have five or more of these symptoms, you are not enjoying your life right now. You can progress from here on in by seeking out a professional to lean on during this difficult time. Do it now!

✦ *Do any necessary grief work.* Depression can stem from grief following a major loss. Whether the loss is small or great, when we fight the grieving process, we prolong depression. Instead of rebelling against this normal, human condition that even the strongest, smartest, and most spiritual people go through, why not join a grief support group?

Community bulletin boards in newspapers list dozens of public support groups for practically every type of loss imaginable. Look for a group, and force yourself to attend at least one meeting. After that, you'll probably go back willingly. Can't find a group that fits your situation? Attend a grief group anyway (many issues related to grief support apply across the board), or start your own by calling a local reporter and telling her your story.

+ ***Eat a nutritionally balanced diet.*** Sometimes, depression stems from vitamin or mineral deficiencies. Researchers at McGill University discovered that some depression may be a result of folic acid deficiencies. The researchers gave depressed subjects 200 mg of folic acid daily and found that their depression eased as a result (although in studies like this, sometimes the nurturing and attention of the researchers—even in well-controlled studies—can elevate the subjects' mood). Still, many studies point to the necessity of taking care of one's body. It's the self-loving thing to do.

+ ***Write down your feelings in a personal journal.*** Sometimes, depression is triggered by confusion or conflicted feelings. When you work through your thoughts on paper, though, the illogical concepts creating the confusion sometimes leap off the page! When "journaling," release any concerns about grammar, punctuation, or spelling. Just let your most vulnerable and honest feelings flow through your pen, and you'll be amazed by the satisfying results.

+ ***Exercise.*** This is definitely one of the best depression-beating techniques I know of. Many studies show that any exercise you do—walking, running, riding your bicycle—will elevate your mood. You're not only creating physical fitness, you're also creating psychological fitness![3]

In one dramatic study, clinically depressed subjects were divided into three groups where they received one of the following treatments for ten weeks: aerobics, relaxation exercises, or no treatment at all. Subjects who aerobically exercised had significantly higher reductions in their depression compared to the other two groups.[4]

AFFIRMATIONS FOR DAIRY CRAVINGS

- ❧ I am safe and secure.

- ❧ I give myself permission to relax.

- ❧ All my needs are taken care of, right now.

- ❧ It's okay for me to let my guard down.

- ❧ I allow my true self to shine through.

SALTY SNACK FOODS:
STRESS, ANGER, AND ANXIETY

A re you a stress eater? Do you munch more when you're under the gun as a result of career, financial, or family pressures? In the Chapter 3 quiz, did you score high in the "Stress Eater" section?

If you answered yes to these questions, then it's also likely that you crave or overeat crispy snack foods such as potato chips, popcorn, and crackers. The crunchy textures provide a cathartic outlet for all the tension held in the jaw. They act like a punching bag! We take our tension and anger out on every crispy bite. Even the crunching sound is reassuring, reminding us of our power as we crush every morsel with our teeth.

Stress Eating

Do Stress Eaters consume more food than other people? Or are they just experiencing more stress?

One study reported that adolescent overeaters had experienced 250 times more life-stress events (such as "parents divorced;" "moved to a new city;" etc.) than adolescents who ate normally.[1]

Studies with rats also confirm the greater life stress theory. One researcher compared the eating habits and weight gain patterns of rats placed under stress, to rats not under stress. This researcher created stress by pinching the rat's tail six times per day (ouch!).

The rats under stress often went on all-out eating binges, and gained an average of 63 grams. The stress-free rats ate normally and only put on 17 grams of weight.[2]

In a similar study with humans (no, they weren't pinched), subjects were given some type of almost impossibly difficult task to perform. That would put most of us under stress, don't you agree? The subjects also had free access to snack foods. As the amount of their stress increased, so did the amount of snack food the subjects consumed.[3]

Women tend to stress-eat more than men, according to researcher Richard Straub of the University of Michigan. Straub asked groups of men and women to watch a movie designed to elicit stressful feelings, as well as a soothing travel film. During the stressful film, men ate less, while the women ate more. The men's eating increased during the travel film (maybe the thought of traveling is more stressful to men?). Straub concluded that many women unnaturally restrict their eating in order to stay thin. But under stress, they cave in and indulge in eating.

Why Do We Stress-Eat?

There are two main theories that explain why we eat more during stressful times:

1. *The Distraction Theory.* When we've got a million things on our mind—the boss, the bills, the kids—our attention is distracted. We become less in-tune with our body, so we are less aware of internal cues of hunger and satiation. When we're stressed, we engage in "automatic eating" (see Chapter 9), and we are less apt to notice when our stomach is quite full.[4]

2. *The Opiate Theory.* Under stress, our bodies produce pain-killing opiates. These opiates appear to stimulate overeating. Researchers have eliminated stress-eating in rats by injecting

them with an opiate-blocking drug called "Naloxone." [5] I have seen this same drug successfully reduce drug and alcohol cravings, probably for the same reasons it blocks stress-eating behaviors.

Salty Cravings

There is nothing inherently wrong with craving salt, since sodium is necessary for survival. I remember a boy I went to school with—his mother had him on a sodium-free diet for some exotic health reason. His personality markedly changed by the second day of his no-salt diet. On the third day, maybe because of all the now-tempting smells of the normally not-so-tempting cafeteria lunches, David fainted in the lunchroom. I remember the school nurse explaining that David's too-stringent diet was responsible for his lost consciousness.

All animals have an innate drive to seek salt. Anyone who has worked with farm animals knows that a "salt lick"—a large block of salt—is as much a part of the farm environment as hay and manure.

Our bodies seek a homeostasis of the blood-to-salt ratios in our bodies. If we stop eating salt, our bodies react by expelling water so we can maintain those same ratios. This mechanism is deadly accurate—if we completely eliminated sodium from our diets, eventually we would die of dehydration. We *need* salt for survival.[6]

Sometimes, as was the case with my school chum David, cravings for sodium and salt are physically based. Studies show that animals go to remarkable lengths to replenish their sodium needs.

For example, porcupines have strong needs for dietary sodium. During the winter, when available vegetation provides insufficient salt, porcupines literally risk their lives to fulfill their salt quotients. At this time of the year, only two sources of salt exist: the sides of barns that have salt left over from winter snows, and roads that have salt thrown on them to relieve icy conditions. Porcupines face the danger presented by trucks, cars, and farmers with shotguns in order to lick salt off of roadsides and barns.[7] (Makes our trips to 7-11 for a bag of Doritos look pretty tame, doesn't it?)

The human craving for salt first appears around four months of age. Prior to that time, infants show no preferences for salt, probably because their taste buds haven't yet developed enough to distinguish salty flavors.[8]

Crunchy Cravings

Think of an animal gnawing away at a bone, and you'll have an accurate mental picture of what a craving for crunchy foods is like. Whether you're yearning for a celery stick or a potato chip, the underlying reason is the same: there's a biological and psychological need to crunch and chew.

One of the primary reasons that diets fail is they don't offer enough crunchy foods to create satiation. All animals, humans included, have a physiological need to chew a certain number of times every day. Eat a bland, soft diet, and you'll feel dissatisfied. That's why most of us can't stick to cottage cheese and yogurt-types of diets. Our teeth feel unfulfilled!

Although our prehistoric ancestors felt a need to crunch on bones to sharpen their teeth, the modern basis of crunchy cravings has to do with 20th-century stress. Your boss yells at you. The account falls through. Your goals are unmet. All of these stressors eat away at you, making you, in turn, want to gnaw away at something crunchy.

A pretzel. Some popcorn. Taco chips. Intuitively, you know that crunching into a food that provides resistance for your teeth will be oh-so-satisfying. Like beating up a punching bag, you can take your frustration and stress out on the "prey" in your mouth. Read about my client Bradley's crunch-craving predicament:

> A patrol cop assigned to cover some of the roughest
> streets in Southern California, he worked the late shift

pulling over drunks and criminals. Bradley's job was stressful, through and through.

Imagine yourself driving a police car and spotting an intoxicated driver. You turn on your lights and siren, pulling the driver over. You exit your car, unsure whether you'll be shot, or abused verbally. Invariably, the drunken driver chooses the latter means of confrontation, rebelling against your authority and power. At moments like that, you wonder what your motivation was for working on the police force.

After unsettling evenings such as these, Bradley would return home at 1:00 a.m. every morning. His wife and children would be asleep, so his company consisted of early-morning television shows and a big bag of potato chips or pretzels. His weight increased by 25 pounds within one year.

"I know I'm eating chips and pretzels to calm down when I get home from work," Bradley told me. "But what else can I do? Should I drink myself to sleep?"

Tension, such as Bradley's, is the third fattening feeling that leads to emotional overeating. Fear, Anger, Tension and Shame (FATS) are extremely uncomfortable to face. We eat to feel better, to help defuse our powerful emotions, and to try and pep up our energy levels. As I've mentioned previously, overeating is rarely in response to a physical need for hunger. It is, instead, a reaction to emotional pain.

Crunching Away at Anger

In addition to tension, we crave crunchy foods when anger becomes overwhelming. Underneath potato chip-eating binges is a monumental fury that is daunting. Many of my clients acknowledge this underlying anger. My client Cindy comes to mind:

The pretty young mother of three could feel the anger building inside of her—"It's like there's a volcano inside of me, ready to erupt."

Yet, that awareness of the anger wasn't enough. Cindy was petrified that if she let loose her anger, she'd behave destructively. "It feels like, if I let out my anger, I'd end up tearing all the walls of this building down. I'd scream at my husband, and I might even hit my kids. I'd slap my boss for being such a jerk. I don't think I'd feel better after destroying everything valuable in my life!"

Cindy felt she had an all-or-nothing choice. Either she held her anger at bay by constantly munching on crackers and popcorn, *or* she'd pummel everyone in her life. No wonder she chose to repress her anger! Her black-and-white belief system led her to believe she was choosing the lesser of two evils.

Cindy and I discussed other options for letting off steam. The most effective, but admittedly most difficult, route when dealing with anger is to heal the source of the problem. In Cindy's case, she was angry at her family and boss for "taking advantage of how nice a person I am."

She described how her husband and kids never helped with the cooking, cleaning, or shopping; how her boss expected her to work overtime, without advance notice, extra pay, or even a "Thank you." And how her co-workers manipulated her into completing their work. Cindy's self-portrait was that of a "martyr-victim."

According to Dr. Helene Parker, author of *If This Is Love, Why Do I Feel So Bad?*, the martyr-victim appears to be at the mercy of others. But in reality, the martyr-victim is a controlling and self-centered individual. Dr. Parker writes: "A common outcome of self-centeredness is 'The Martyr Syndrome.' This occurs when a person doesn't pursue happiness, then blames others for the resulting unhappiness. The Martyr tries to elicit guilt from others to feel in control, needed, and loved. Unfortunately, The Martyr Syndrome never results in good feelings or positive love."[9]

This explanation described Cindy's situation perfectly, so I worked with her to resolve the sources of her stress. We worked on basic, but productive, solutions for her problems, such as creating chores lists for her kids and having her initiate discussions with her husband regarding the need to share responsibility. I encouraged Cindy to behave assertively with her boss and co-workers. Although she feared the consequences of saying no, Cindy was very pleased with the results of her new behavior.

"I had thought that asking for help was a sign of weakness. I was afraid that other people would reject me if I wasn't 'perfect' or if I didn't play Miss Caretaker all the time," she explained.

Cindy remembered how difficult it was to change a lifetime habit of pretending to always be happy. "In the beginning, it was terrifying to tell other people what I really thought. I felt like my husband would leave me and I'd lose my job. The irony was, though, if I hadn't shared my opinions, I would have eventually left my marriage and job. The situations were unbearable, and I was miserable! Now, I'm much more honest with everybody about what my limits are. And that feels damn good for a change!"

In Cindy's case, all the introspective therapy in the world would not have helped her as much as the seemingly simple course we took: taking action. Cindy had to push herself to verbalize her need for help. Once she got a positive response from her husband, kids, co-workers, and boss, it was infinitely easier to speak up the second, third, and fourth time. She gained respect

and assistance and, in turn, felt little need to continually chomp on snack foods.

Self-Directed Anger Equals Depression

You've probably heard the expression, "Depression is anger
turned inward." It's a simplistic statement, yet in many cases of depression it is entirely true. Women, in particular, have been so-
cialized that expressing anger is *bad*. They learn young that the way
to please Mommy, Daddy, and teacher is to silently smile and never,
ever rock the boat. As young women, they learn that boys are more
attracted to them if they smile instead of frown.

Women never learn how to effectively manage this most powerful emotion. So they opt to stuff it down and pretend it doesn't
exist — as if it's a sign of weakness to feel anger!

Yet anger is a normal, natural emotion in both sexes. As I wrote
in my book, *Losing Your Pounds of Pain*, anger is the number-one
emotion triggering compulsive overeating. We are angry when we
are born, due to the trauma of birth. We are angry as babies when
we feel hungry, thirsty, wet, or tired. As children, we feel anger toward classmates who hit us, or little brothers who steal our toys.

In its pure state, anger is the fuel of the exquisitely beautiful emotion we call "passion." Have you ever talked or acted passionately
about some cause you've deeply believed in? Have you ever been
moved by a passionate speaker sincerely committed to his or her
cause? Think of Martin Luther King, John F. Kennedy, and Glo-
ria Steinem. Their impassioned and compelling speeches —
whether you agree with the sentiments expressed or not — are prime
examples of the awe-inspiring beauty of anger that is directed towards something meaningful.

The ugly side of anger occurs when it is held in. That's when
anger turns into a rotted, decrepit version of itself. Anger, repressed,
turns into resentment, bitterness, frustration, and depression.
Contrast the mental image of the passionate speaker with an elderly

person, bitter and frustrated because of missed opportunities. Which image would you prefer for yourself?

Fat and Furious

Author Dr. Judi Hollis writes poignantly about how food masks anger. At her inpatient eating disorder center, many of the patients enter with a forced "everything's just fine" grin. But in reality, everything isn't just fine for these patients—that's why they are seeking some assistance with their emotional pain. But because food is such an effective temporary emotional anesthesia, these women can't admit the depth of their pain to themselves.

In *Fat and Furious: Women and Food Obsession,* Hollis describes the early days of a patient's treatment:

> Most of my patients are admitted to the hospital with a diagnosis of depression. Of course! Who wouldn't be depressed by the hopeless cycle of gaining and losing hundreds of pounds. Many sense that they are depressed because they've lived so far from their true heart's message. They are so out of touch with spirit, so lost from their inner selves, that despite their sometimes superhuman functioning, they have become extremely depressed.
>
> For many, that depression won't surface until their fourth or sixth day of treatment. That's when sugar withdrawals are the worst. Countless patients enter treatment full of smiles and gratitude, telling us how sweet the intake counselor was, how much they like the nursing staff, how they can't wait to get up early for exercise and meditation.
>
> But let's face it, most of them have been eating their "last supper" for at least a week before they come, so those smiles are really plastered on a walking glucose bottle. That draining bottle starts hitting bottom around the fourth day, and a raging, fuming, hostile combatant wakes up. Then she hates the nursing staff,

feeling "they're all out to get me," and has a mile-long list of grievances at how inefficiently our unit is run.

But as she weathers this storm of rage, it passes, and within a few days she is embarrassed and apologetic. No need for either. It's the nature of the beast. Depression is anger turned inward....[10]

9 WAYS TO REDUCE SALTY SNACK FOOD CRAVINGS

When those frustrating cravings urge you to eat chips, crackers, popcorn, or pretzels, here are some appetite-reducing strategies:

1. *Crunch on crisp vegetables dipped in low-calorie, fat-free salad dressing.* Instead of potato chips, go for carrot sticks decadently dripping with flavorful dressing. Keep carrot and celery sticks, as well as broccoli and cauliflower florets, handy in the refrigerator so you'll have no excuse to bypass this healthful alternative.

2. *Ask yourself, "Am I really craving crunchy, salty foods, or am I instead craving fat?"* Do you dream of crispy french fries, greasy potato chips, or freshly fried onion rings? If nothing but a high-fat or fried crunchy snack will do, then your cravings may have less to do with crunchiness or saltiness, and more to do with fat content. In that case, follow the suggestions in Chapter 21.

3. *If you're angry at someone else, realize that it makes no sense to punish yourself by overeating unhealthful foods.* You're devouring those salty, greasy potato chips, so you must know that you are the only person who will suffer the effects of feeling sluggish, bloated, and overweight. Take out your anger in healthy and productive ways (such as exercise), instead of attacking yourself.

4. *Address the source of your stress, tension, or anxiety.* When it comes to dealing with cravings, the best solution is to heal the source of the problem. What is causing your stress? What steps—even small ones—can you take to relieve some of it? Even though those steps may seem a bit frightening, push yourself to resolve some of your uneasy feelings right now. Deep down, you already know what those steps entail, but you are afraid of the consequences. You're afraid that you'll make things worse, instead of better. Visualize what a better life would look like, and tell others what you will and won't accept. You'll be doing yourself an incredible favor, and you'll feel empowered right after you take positive action.

5. *Sprinkle a minimal amount of salt on top of foods after you serve them, instead of cooking salt into the foods.* You tend to taste salt more if it is on the surface of food, rather than cooked as one of the food's ingredients. That is because salt loses its salty taste—but none of its sodium content—during the cooking process.

    In one study, subjects were given salt-free foods as well as unlimited access to salt shakers. The subjects added only 20 percent of the amount of salt that normally would have been included in each food's cooking ingredients.[11] One researcher concluded that, when it comes to salt cravings, "... the saltiness the mouth experiences, not the amount of sodium actually ingested, is responsible for how much someone prefers a salty food."[12]

6. *Exercise!* It will make you feel *much* better in the long run than a bowl of popcorn, chips, or pretzels. Are you ready to blow your lid at your roommate, husband, or boss? Instead of opening the cupboard or refrigerator door, walk out the front door and go for a long, fast-paced walk. Have a long mental talk with yourself about your problem, your feelings, and possible solutions.

7. *Throw out, or remove yourself from, crunchy snack foods while you deal with the source of your stress or anger.* One time, I was angry because my future mother-in-law had gone to visit my fiancé's ex-girlfriend. My head told me, "There's no reason to be jealous," but my heart hurt with fear-based feelings such as, "She likes the ex-girlfriend better than she likes me." While trying to reconcile these conflicting thoughts and feelings, I was standing next to a bowl of party snack crackers. I was shocked to discover that I was absent-mindedly gnawing away at the crackers. They didn't taste all that great, but the texture provided a small outlet for my frustration. Once I saw what I was doing, I took evasive action and poured the crackers into the garbage. I knew that until I resolved my feelings, it was self-loving to remove all sources of temptation. (P.S. I resolved the issue by discussing the matter with my fiancé and his mother.)

8. *Call someone.* Talking to a counselor, close friend, or relative will relieve some of that pent-up anger and help you feel validated. You'll also be able to come up with some possible solutions, which will make you feel more hopeful about your situation.

9. *Write down your feelings.* A 1994 study of 535 women by University of Tennessee's Dr. Sandra Thomas concluded that women who wrote down their angry thoughts in a journal were among the healthiest in her study. They were less prone to overeating, headaches, or stomachaches than women who yelled when they were angry, or who totally repressed their anger. Putting my feelings into words is my own personal choice for dealing with emotional upsets. I always feel much better after I note down every thought and emotion that I'm aware of on a piece of paper or on my computer screen. I've

never used a formal "journal" or diary, but many of my clients like them. The beauty of "journaling" is that there are no rules governing right or wrong ways to write. It's not like being in English 101. Instead, you simply get out a piece of paper and start writing everything you think and feel. Don't worry about spelling, neatness, grammar, or any "writing rules." Just write, and you'll feel infinitely better about your situation.

AFFIRMATIONS FOR SNACK FOOD CRAVINGS

- All tension has left my body.
- I forgive myself and others.
- I give myself permission to let go of blame.
- I take excellent care of myself.
- My friends are loving, thoughtful, and giving.

SPICY FOODS:
THE DRIVE FOR EXCITEMENT

D o you season your foods before tasting them? Is your food philosophy, "The spicier the better"? Do you adore Mexican, Thai, or spicy Chinese food, and abhor bland foods such as English or traditional American dishes?

Food probably isn't the only area of your life that you prefer spicy. You may also crave excitement and high intensity in your work, love, and play life as well. If you aren't getting enough thrills, you may convert that frustration into intense cravings for spicy foods.

Psychologist, researcher, and author Bernard Lyman describes "sensation seekers" as people who "seem to need extra excitement and often enjoy taking risks. [Sensation seeking] is measured by answers to questions involving choices between high and low activity or between danger and security.... Sensation-seeking has been correlated with several behavior patterns including delinquency. The assumption is that lawbreaking and the danger of being caught give these persons the extra excitement they crave."[1]

Several researchers have correlated "sensation seeking" with cravings for spicy, crunchy, or sour foods; gourmet foods, and unusual, exotic foods. Another study concluded that overweight women were particularly prone to cravings for intensely flavored foods.[2] Spicy Food Cravers have strong desires for novelty and change—kind of like "pushing the envelope" via exotic eating experiences.

Spicy Oriental Food

Monosodium glutamate (MSG) is a stimulant liberally used in most Chinese food, unless you ask the chef to leave it out (even then, I always wonder …). MSG is a sodium salt of an amino acid, known to amplify the flavor of whatever food it's added to. It also has its own unique taste.

Have you ever left a Chinese restaurant and felt odd? Sometimes, people joke about being hungry within an hour of eating Chinese food. Such jokes usually contain a kernel of truth, don't they? Part of the hour-later hunger stems from the low-fat content of Chinese food. If you are accustomed to a high-fat diet, you won't feel full or satisfied at first when you switch to low-fat foods. It takes about a month to adapt to such a diet.

But another part of post-Chinese restaurant hunger is emotional, an attempt to feel better. MSG creates reactions known as "Chinese Restaurant Syndrome," or "Kwok's Disease." Symptoms can be intense or mild, and include headaches, nausea, giddiness, perspiration, and facial or neck muscle tightening.[3] Have you ever experienced any of these symptoms?

MSG acts as a stimulant. One study showed that, in extremely high doses, MSG can stimulate brain neurons so much that it could result in death.[4] Thrill-seekers who thrive on stimulation are attracted to Chinese food for the sensations that MSG and hot spices induce.

People who are resentful and stressed because their life is all work and no play, and especially those who crave *thrilling* types of fun, often crave spicy food mixed with nuts. In Chinese food that translates into kung pao chicken, a mixture of Szechwan-style hot peppers, chicken, and peanuts in a slightly sweet sauce. It is poured over ultra-crispy vegetables, which soothes the stressed, frustrated, or resentful person's need to gnaw.

Individuals who thrive on high-adrenaline lifestyles — especially entertainment-industry professionals, stockbrokers, and salespersons—often crave spicy noodle Oriental food, such as traditional Thai dishes. The peppers pump you up, while the noodles calm you down—a food that's a perfect metaphor for this type of person's roller-coaster lifestyle.

An interesting study was once conducted at Oriental restaurants by a very respected research team. The researchers sat near the door of each restaurant, noting the body size of each patron that entered the establishment. Each patron was categorized as being either "obese" or "non-obese."

Next, the researchers observed which patrons used chopsticks to eat their meals. They found that almost one-fourth of the non-obese, but only 5 percent of the obese, ate their meals with chopsticks. The researchers concluded that the obese wanted to eat bigger mouthfuls than a chopstick allows for.[5]

Spicy Mexican Food

Many spicy Mexican dishes are seasoned with hot chili peppers. These peppers really give Spicy Food Eaters the boost they crave—there's an actual increase in body temperature in response to eating chili peppers.

This body-temperature increase is followed by a cooling-off period, creating a hot-and-cold effect that's useful in extremely hot climates. For Spicy Food Eaters, the body temperature roller-coaster ride is exciting. It simulates an adrenaline burst.[6]

Chili peppers are usually so hot that they painfully burn the mouth. This pain is appealing to some thrill seekers, who require higher-than-normal levels of stimulation. Some Spicy Food Eaters like to prove their toughness, actually engaging in contests to see who can eat the biggest jalapeño pepper without drinking water.

Other people enjoy a more private mouth-burning experience, where the hot sensations trigger adrenaline, hormonal, and opiate reactions in response to the pain. Whenever the body experiences pain, the brain secretes the hormone cortisol (which in synthetic form is called "cortisone," found in the shots that athletes receive for pain). The cortisol flows throughout the body in response to a specific discomfort. In this way, someone who eats a painfully hot chili pepper will be rewarded with an enveloping sensation of pain-numbing cortisol.

By eating hot chilis, Spicy Food Eaters are self-medicating. The question is, are they self-medicating because they are in physical pain, or are they trying to sedate some type of emotional pain?

The Spice/Personality Link

Spicy Food Bingers have personalities that are as strong as the seasonings on their foods! Sometimes, their personalities are over-powering.

Some Spicy Food Bingers have blunted taste buds. Alcohol or excessive smoking compete with their taste buds' abilities to de-tect salty, sour, and spicy tastes. One study found that children of alcoholics have fewer taste buds than normal, creating a chicken-and-the-egg question.[7] When you have fewer taste buds, you are less sensitive to strong flavors, including the flavors in alcohol. Spicy Food Bingers require more seasoning on their foods just to reach the level most would consider normal.

An acquaintance of mine is a classic Spicy Food Binger. Hank is a professional journalist with a romantic notion of himself as a modern-day Hemingway. As such, Hank stays drunk throughout much of the day. It's no coincidence that he also carries a jar of seasoned salt in his pocket. He is always afraid that the food served at restaurants or at friends' houses won't be spicy enough. So he unabashedly sprinkles liberal helpings of the sea-soned salt on every food placed in front of him. He never pretastes the food to see if it is salty or spicy enough. Hank, with his alcohol-numbed taste buds, always as-sumes that food needs additional seasoning.

Sometimes, Spicy Food cravings are a defense against an overly stimulating lifestyle.

Denise, a woman I once knew, was a petite, blonde highway patrolwoman. The daughter of a police sergeant, Denise decided as a young child that she'd be a law enforcement officer. She felt that her Dad was disappointed that she wasn't a boy. To win his love, Denise played the role of "perfect son." She downplayed her natural beauty and femininity and became an androgenous police officer.

Every day, Denise would face danger inherent in her treacherous job, and she would be filled with heart-pumping adrenaline each time she'd walk to a car she'd pulled over. The price of pleasing her father was quite high, and it wasn't exactly paying off as planned, either! Her Dad still hadn't said, "I'm proud of you," the words she so longed to hear. Maybe if she got a promotion at the department...

Denise dealt with her overstimulated life through the use of Tabasco sauce. She poured the hot sauce onto everything she ate—even ice cream! For Denise, this spicy condiment clearly acted as an anesthetic. She was triggering her brain chemicals to alleviate her emotional pain by purposely creating physical pain in the form of mouth burn! Kind of like an intuitive acupuncture technique, wouldn't you say?

Spicy Food Bingers are often very successful people. Since they love the rush involved in taking huge risks, these are the people who are usually the high rollers when it comes to their careers. Those who win are often Spicy Food Bingers such as Phil Donahue, Geraldo Rivera, and Sally Jessy Raphael. How do I know that? Well, I analyzed all three of their food-craving personalities on national television. Many people who are hugely successful in volatile industries, such as the media, are Spicy Food Bingers.

Enthusiasm: The Lasting High

Those individuals who are quite successful, who enjoy long-lasting success, are usually motivated by their own natural source of jet fuel. This outcome results from paying attention to the gut feelings that tell them which career and life path to follow. When your actions resonate in harmony with your inner direction and beliefs, you have access to unlimited energy and enthusiasm. You wake up in the morning rarin' to go!

Those who are selling themselves short, who engage in activities they know are meaningless or dishonest, feel drained and lethargic. They may seek excitement in artificial or synthetic ways, such as Spicy Foods.

Excitement is a physical high stemming from adrenaline. It is short-lived and ultimately very draining. Enthusiasm, on the other hand, provides a lasting high and results in increased energy. Excitement is drawn from external sources, such as eating spicy foods, going on a roller coaster, or being in a dangerous situation. Enthusiasm comes from internal sources, such as taking steps toward fulfilling your dreams.

Spices That Block Pain

Really hot spices encourage the brain to release pain-relieving chemicals that bathe and numb the entire body. It's a natural way to seek emotional anesthesia, but it's still a Band-Aid, a temporary measure. Ask yourself, "What's really bothering me?" and "What do I really want and need?"

Once the answers surface, it's a part of self-responsibility and self-love to take the steps toward fulfilling these desires. Even before you achieve your ultimate goals, you'll feel so much better!

Knowing that you are progressing in the direction of your dreams is a therapeutic feeling that will relieve any desire to self-medicate with chili peppers.

AFFIRMATIONS FOR SPICY FOOD CRAVINGS

- Time is an abundant and unlimited resource.
- I have enough time to take care of all my needs.
- I am fulfilling all of my dreams right now.
- I have the intelligence and creativity to accomplish everything I set my mind to.
- I listen to, and follow, my inner voice.
- I deserve to have the life I desire.
- I make sure I meet all of my needs for excitement and stimulation.

LIQUID CRAVINGS:
UP-AND-DOWN ENERGY CYCLES

S ometimes, people find that they have a Constant Craving for liquids. As is the case with solid foods, most beverages contain mood-altering properties that appeal to those seeking immediate shelter from emotional pain. The three primary liquids craved are diet sodas, coffee, and alcohol.

Diet Colas and Eating Binges

I was always amazed by how many of my clients carried a can of diet cola into their initial therapy session with me. Gabrielle was a typical example:

> The pretty brunette shyly entered my office carrying a bright red-and-white aluminum can of diet cola. She sipped it as she answered my initial questions about why she'd come to see me. The sips turned to gulps as Gabrielle began unpeeling the details of her life.
>
> She'd talk about her on-again-off-again boyfriend, and take a swig. Then she'd discuss her much-divorced mother, and gulp the majority of the can's remaining liquid.
>
> For Gabrielle and most of my other diet cola-swilling clients, the liquid represented a safety valve—something to hang onto that would provide energy and excitement

without the "commitment" of fat or calories. Kind of like
a perfect boyfriend.

Diet cola is one of the favorite stimulants of chronic dieters. I
don't say this as an insult or an accusation, but as an observer of
real life. Plus, I used to be among their ranks! When I was in college, I "used" diet cola—sometimes drinking two liters a day—to
keep me awake while I studied at night. Now, my cravings for cola
are gone. I never drink the stuff, and have probably had one can in
the last five years. I'm happy to report that I don't miss it, either
(in addition, my skin is a lot clearer as a result of having given up
all those artificial chemicals!).

The carbonation in diet colas makes the caffeine and the artificial sweetener, NutraSweet, kick in that much faster. It's a refreshing drink, and it fills you up. Many women use diet cola as a
substitute for meals and sustenance. "I don't need lunch or dinner;
I'll just drink this diet cola," they'll say.

NutraSweet is composed of two amino acids: aspartic acid and
phenylalanine. Both amino acids have a highly stimulating effect
and trigger the production of excitatory neurotransmitters. Aspartic acid, in particular, has been linked to increased stamina and en-
durance, and decreased fatigue. No wonder diet drinks are the
darlings of women on the fast track—all the stimulating ingredients keep them going.

But many studies show that those no-calorie drinks could lead
to high-calorie eating binges later in the day. Sweet Eaters are attracted to a sweet taste, even when sugar isn't the sweetening ingredient. Still other people are highly sensitive to the chemical taste
of artificial sweeteners. They won't eat anything smacking of saccharin or NutraSweet.

However, the majority of Sweet Eaters love a sweet taste, regardless of its source. Several studies have recorded this behavior,
showing that overeating binges often occur in response to ingest-
ing sweet-tasting food. In these studies, overeating was the case

even when the sweetening agent was artificial or dietetic. In fact, some people binge-eat "dietetic" food, overeating so much of it that weight gain, or even obesity, is the result. Several researchers believe that artificial sweeteners stimulate the appetite, and actually *trigger* eating binges! [1]

It makes sense that an artificial sweetener, such as aspartame (marketed as "NutraSweet") could trigger eating binges. As stated earlier, one of the two core ingredients is an amino acid called phenylalanine. It has been marketed as a "natural" sweetener, since amino acids occur naturally in protein products.

However, many people are sensitive to phenylalanine. Perhaps you've noticed little warning labels on the sides of diet cola cans and bottles telling anyone with PKU to avoid drinking the beverage. This term refers to *phenylketonuria,* a malady afflicting about one in every 20,000 children. These children are born without the enzyme necessary to metabolize the amino acid, phenylalanine. Since the child can't metabolize this substance, it accumulates in his or her body, resulting in irreversible and debilitating retardation.

Many people who don't have PKU still experience adverse reactions to this amino acid. There are many documented complaints of people reporting feelings of dizziness, lethargy, jitteryness, or light-headedness following the ingestion of phenylalanine in the form of NutraSweet.[2]

I have found that carbonated beverages, in general, create psychological effects. The carbon monoxide may compete with oxygen, or may speed the effects of caffeine and NutraSweet. Some women have reported panic attacks following undue life stress mixed with drinking a large quantity of diet colas. (The carbonation is suspected of contributing to these attacks.) It is well known, after all, that alcoholic beverages that are carbonated result in faster intoxication than noncarbonated alcoholic beverages.

Colas also reduce your body's magnesium levels, thereby potentially inspiring food cravings. A study conducted by Kenneth Weaver, M.D., at East Tennessee University, found that phosphoric acid in cola binds with, and extracts, the body's magnesium. Each 12-ounce can of cola contains 36 milligrams of phosphoric acid, resulting in the removal of 36 milligrams of magnesium.[3]

If it sounds like I'm building a case against cola (no pun intended!), I'm not. Moderation, in everything, is always the wisest choice.

Coffee Bingeing

Coffee Bingers are invariably trying to invigorate a tired horse—namely, themselves! They are loaded down with unwanted responsibilities, so they attempt to make their energy levels live up to their overly burdened schedules. Instead of listening to their gut feelings—the true source of energy—Coffee Bingers try to artificially elicit enthusiasm for projects they really don't believe in.

Coffee seems to be an acquired taste. Some researchers even believe the appetite for coffee is a conditioned response. Studies show that if we eat or drink a pleasant-tasting food with an unpleasant-tasting food, eventually we will grow to like the unpleasant food.[4] We will associate the unpleasant food with the pleasure we receive from its better-tasting companion.

Researcher A.W. Logue believes that this phenomenon explains how humans develop a taste for coffee and tea, two drinks that she argues are initially unpleasant tasting until we grow accustomed to drinking them. Logue writes: "A new coffee or tea drinker usually adds more palatable substances such as sugar and milk to the beverage. Gradually, as the actual taste of the coffee or tea becomes associated with the taste of the sugar or the milk, the coffee or tea can be drunk with less, and finally no, sugar or milk."[5]

Coffee Bingers usually wake up in the morning dreading the hours ahead. They often hold jobs that don't correspond to their natural interests and desires. Their motivation to work is usually based on fears of financial ruin, so excessive coffee consumption helps them get through the day.

The Coffee Binger may have gut feelings about what career would truly be interesting and worthwhile, but fears and self-doubts stand in the way. After years of relying on their unhealthy motivational "tools," Coffee Bingers find themselves addicted to fears of financial problems, as well as to coffee.

Gut feelings encompass detailed road maps of the career path you are supposed to follow. This career is normally something that fascinates and naturally motivates you, one that will give you freedom from financial strain and which will help other people. Meditation and quiet contemplation can give you a great deal of direction. I really believe that if each of us concentrated on developing a life purpose that was truly meaningful, the world as a whole would benefit.

The Appeal of Alcohol

Have you ever had one alcoholic beverage and felt incredibly good? Then you have another drink and you lose that great feeling? You're not alone. Alcohol, in small doses, acts as a stimulant. But, in greater amounts, alcohol changes its tune and becomes a depressant.

Sugar cravers — those who crave candy or cookies — are sometimes alcohol cravers as well. This is no accident. Sugar and alcohol are almost identical in their molecular structure. Just as sugar triggers eating binges, so too does alcohol.

Those who drink beer and wine are often seeking a stimulant effect, even as they crave stress management. Both of these beverages contain large amounts of tyramine, which is created by the fermentation process. Tyramine raises blood pressure and stimulates the production of the brain chemical, noradrenaline. These drinks provide a kick that has nothing to do with their alcohol content!

Alcohol also temporarily raises the brain's serotonin level, which raises the question of whether drinking is a self-medicating behavior. Serotonin, as you'll recall, is crucial to a feeling of well-being. Some studies indicate that chronic drinkers may have lower serotonin levels than social or non-drinkers. Perhaps they are trying to drink "liquid" serotonin. Unfortunately, as you'll read, alcohol's serotonin-boosting effect is short-lived. In the long run, excessive alcohol consumption depletes serotonin production.[6]

The emotional issues most strongly associated with alcohol cravings include:

+ Anger

+ Depression

+ Grief

+ Loneliness

+ Shame

Yet, as most of us know, alcohol cravings and alcohol overindulgence can amplify our negative emotions. As we've read, alcohol acts as a depressant. It can also work against our desires for healthful lifestyles. While alcohol in moderation isn't a problem for most people (aside from recovering alcoholics who need to completely abstain), excessive alcohol actually leads to food cravings and weight gain. As I wrote in my book, *Losing Your Pounds of Pain:*

> The alcoholic body has a difficult time distinguishing between alcohol and sugar, and feels the need to binge on one or both substances. This makes sense when you consider that alcohol is created out of food: wine is fermented fruit; beer is made from grain; vodka from potatoes, and so on.
>
> Studies of brain chemistry in alcoholics also point to physiological causes for alcoholism. We know that there are genetic

predispositions toward alcoholism; in other words, you can inherit the desire to abuse alcohol. Several researchers have discovered that the brain chemical, serotonin, may be depleted in alcoholic brains. As you may recall, when serotonin is low, you feel lethargic or irritable. Researchers believe alcoholics may be self-medicating, attempting to compensate for the depleted serotonin by getting drunk.

Unfortunately, alcohol abuse results in further serotonin depletion. Serotonin is a chemical that forms in the brain as you sleep. Your brain doesn't store the substance; it must be created from scratch every night. What happens is this: Your body converts a body substance, melatonin, into the brain chemical, serotonin, during the Rapid Eye Movement (REM) phase of the nightly sleep cycle. If your REM sleep cycle is interrupted, you won't create enough serotonin. And then you'll wake up feeling groggy.

Excessive consumption of alcohol and other drugs interferes with REM sleep. If you drink too much before bed, you won't get enough REM sleep, and you'll wake up with a hangover from depleted serotonin. Those suffering from the pain/pound link may notice they crave carbohydrates (breads, sweets, and starchy foods) when their serotonin is low.

Even worse, alcohol interferes with weight-loss efforts. First alcohol is very fattening. Second, alcohol slows the body down. It is a depressant. But whoops! It especially slows down metabolism, the rate at which your body burns calories. So, not only does alcohol ADD calories to your body, but it also makes you burn those calories at a slower rate.

Finally—and you're probably aware of this from personal experience—if you've been drinking or you're hungover, you're less likely to exercise. Even though a workout would probably make you feel much better, when you're tired or irritated, you just want to relax. So, you burn even fewer calories because your energy level is low.[7]

Love Cravings and Liquid Cravings

Cravings for love can also trigger binge-drinking on alcohol and diet cola. One study asked subjects to imagine what they'd like to eat or drink when they were experiencing feelings of love or affection. The number-one answer given? Wine. The researchers explained the wine-love link in this way: "... the largest preference for alcohol was not during anger, frustration, or depression when it is supposedly used to alleviate the feelings, but during 'love-affection,' when individuals reported using wine with meals to prolong the mood."[8]

Diet drinks may also correspond to cravings for romance. As you've just read, phenylalanine is one of the two ingredients of aspartame, or NutraSweet. Some studies suggest that phenylalanine may encourage the brain to produce phenylethylamine (PEA), the amphetamine substance correlated with feelings of romantic love. So diet soft drinks may be functioning in a similar manner to chocolate-bingeing. The underlying drive may be a desire for the brain chemistry associated with romantic love.[9]

Two Other Natural Sources of Energy

You have unlimited energy when you live in harmony with your deepest beliefs. The other two natural sources of incredible energy are exercise and water.

Throughout this book, you may have noticed how I've been encouraging you to exercise. I'm not trying to act like a high school gym coach; I just know from first-hand experience the tremendous cure-all effect of exercise. On those days when you feel tired, depressed, hungover, premenstrual, or just plain miserable, give exercise a try. Do something aerobic for at least 15 minutes, where you can work up a good sweat. Your aerobic level of activity will have you breathing hard enough so you can't sing (anything less isn't strenuous enough), but not so hard that you can't talk (which would put you into the anaerobic level where fat is not being burned).

So many studies underscore the remarkable therapeutic benefits of exercise. I have been a mental and physical health researcher for years, regularly scouring the journals of medical and psychological organizations. Exercise is one of the few topics that usually inspires a consensus among researchers. With few exceptions, exercise is always beneficial.

As for the benefits associated with water, the next time your energy level is low, wait a minute before taking a caffeine break. Try water instead. Water is refreshing and rejuvenating and is a remarkable source of natural energy. Make water a special drink by serving it to yourself in a beautiful crystal glass, complete with a lemon slice!

Affirmations for Liquid Cravings

🐸 I have enough energy to accomplish all my desires.

🐸 I ask, and receive, the help of others.

🐸 I love myself just as I am now.

🐸 I accept all that is good in my life.

🐸 I release the need to be in a hurry.

🐸 I forgive all my past sources of pain, and allow pleasure to enter my being now.

🐸 I can relax and trust my intuition.

🐸 It's okay to let down my guard and defenses.

🐸   🐸   🐸

NUTS AND PEANUT BUTTER: CRAVINGS FOR FUN

In our stressed-out, time-constrained world, there seems to be little room for relaxation and pleasure. Yet, all creatures need fun. Just look at your pets at home, or the animals on television documentaries. They all play! Fun and play are as natural as breathing and drinking. We often try to put this basic human need on the back burner, hoping it will go away. But, like all repressed desires and emotions, ignoring it doesn't make it go away. Instead, its appeal just gets stronger.

Nut cravings are an expression of unmet needs for fun and pleasure. The chemicals inherent in nuts, as well as the textures associated with them, tend to soothe fun-deprived individuals.

In my book, *Yo-Yo Relationships*[1], I discuss why I believe fun is a necessity, not a luxury. When we repress the need for fun, we experience (seriously!) "Fun-Deprivation Syndrome." This is similar to burn-out, and its symptoms include: feeling tired, cranky, and irritable that your life is out of whack; and forgetting what "fun" means.

There are many rationalizations for excluding fun from your life. Among the common statements I've heard people use to explain away their need for recreation include:

— "I need to devote time and energy to my children and husband."
— "First I have to accomplish my goals, then I'll have fun."
— "I can't be that selfish."
— "Other people may need to have fun, but I'm above all that!"

Fun-deprived people often use nuts as an immediate source for inducing pleasure chemicals in the brain, as well as an outlet for frustration or a source of comfort. Some people who live overly stressed lifestyles devoid of any fun are lacking enthusiasm. They are burned out and in need of an injection of amusement and gaiety in their lives. Nuts offer this outlet. Cashews and peanuts contain large amounts of tyrosine, which is a vasoactive substance that raises blood pressure.[2]

Nuts also contain pyrazine, which triggers the pleasure center of the brain.[3] The mere smell of a freshly opened can of mixed nuts or a jar of peanut butter provides a strong whiff of pyrazine and a hefty dose of pleasure chemicals. Many of my clients binge-eat nuts due to their unfulfilled desires for pure fun and enjoyment:

— Nuts are high in fat, and fat masks feelings of emptiness, loneliness, worry, or discontent. Neal was very worried because his company was undergoing a merger. He was working long, hard hours to prove his worth to the outside consultants who were trying to decide who should stay and who should go. Neal's job insecurities, time constrictions, and lack of recreational outlets created the perfect climate for his daily binges on peanuts.

— Nuts are also crunchy, perfect for the Stress Eater. Frustrated in her job, Henrietta found herself "picking" at the sunflower seeds she had in her desk drawer. Handful by handful, she'd scoop the oily, salty nuts into her mouth. As Henrietta ground the sunflower seeds in her mouth, she felt more satisfied with her situation. In truth, the seeds were an emotional outlet for Henrietta, allowing her to gnaw away at her dissatisfaction with her career.

— Nuts can also be creamy smooth, perfect for the comfort-seeker. LuAnne's craving was for creamy peanut butter, as well as soft peanut butter cookies. She couldn't get enough! Her food-craving analysis confirmed that LuAnne was afraid to relax and have fun. She feared that her husband would judge her as lazy or indulgent if she goofed off for a while during the day. These fears triggered her compulsion to feverishly work around the house. She craved, and ate, a lot of peanut butter to ease her self-pity over having a life devoid of fun.

— Nuts can also be highly seasoned, sometimes spicy hot, perfect for the Spicy Thrill Seeker. Robert loved to eat Cajun-style peanuts, the spicier and saltier the better. He crunched into each bite, enjoying the burning flavor and sensation. This craving shows a high level of emotional pain. There is a real sense of being deprived of life's pleasure, along with an anger associated with missing out on all the fun. Spicy Nut Cravers would really benefit from injecting any amount of fun possible into their lives.

— Nuts also come in honey-sweetened styles, perfect for the Sugar Binger. Wendy felt drained by her lifestyle of all work and no play. She was definitely a "Superwoman" who did too much, relying on coffee, chocolate, and honey-roasted peanuts to get her through the day. Her cravings for nuts signaled Fun Deprivation Syndrome, and her anger toward the situation manifested itself in her cravings for crunchy nuts, which she'd munch on continually. The honey-sweetened coating helped boost her flagging energy. For Wendy, her draining, fun-deprived life was an unfortunate choice — she had enough money to be able to take a vacation or start a hobby. Yet Wendy didn't believe fun was a worthwhile pursuit. So she ate instead.

— Nuts can also be combined with chocolate, in either crunchy or creamy forms. Chocolate-covered nuts provided an outlet for Tricia, who was frustrated and angry about her boring love life. Tricia wanted to go dancing and have nights of enjoyment with her boyfriend—that signified love and romance to her. However, her boyfriend preferred to spend evenings and weekends watching sports on television.

— Peanut butter and chocolate cup cravings are really a craving for hugs and comfort due to a love life that lacks fun. My client Anita also craved having fun with her husband. But instead of feeling anger and frustration, Anita was usually depressed, blaming the lack of fun in her life on her and her husband's tight budget. So, she just kept eating those peanut butter cups.

Nuts can also be combined with dairy products, such as ice cream, for a really emotionally medicating treat. Smooth varieties, such as peanut butter frozen yogurt or ice cream, indicate some depression over the lack of fun. Crunchy varieties, such as almond toffee, signal anger or frustration that life is more work than play.

Fun Is a Necessity, Not a Luxury

As you can probably tell, I'm definitely advocating the injection of regular doses of fun into your life as a step to healing nut cravings. Not only is fun a necessity, it also yields wonderful benefits. When we enjoy ourselves, we feel enthused, alive, energized. Our inner child glows, and we laugh and let go.

As I wrote in my book, *Yo-Yo Relationships*:

> Children naturally have pure fun (as opposed to competitive fun)—just for the thrill, pleasure, and joy. What did you do for fun as a child? When did you feel happiest? If you can't remember, then you might spend some time watching children

play. Notice how they revel—without a sign of embarrassment, reluctance, or guilt—in the pure joy of touching the sky with their feet as they swing, or coaxing a kite higher and higher. Remember when you used to do stuff like that? You haven't outgrown your appetite for fun, any more than you've lost the need to eat and breathe. If anything, we need to laugh *more* now that we're responsibility-laden adults![1]

I also believe that our internal "fun zone" guides us to career paths of prosperity. My own father, Bill Hannan, is a perfect example. He turned his childhood hobby of building balsa wood airplanes into an occupation. Today, my father has written over 15 books on the subject and writes regular columns for *Model Builder* magazine. He's my living example of turning your source of fun into a source of income. Dad has enjoyed perfect health, the ability to work from home, prosperity, fame, and wonderful friendships—all because he followed his heart and did for a living what he would naturally do for free.

Ask yourself: "What is my heart's desire right now?" "If a millionaire would bankroll my wildest dream, what would I do?" "What job would I love to do, even if there was no salary or pay of any kind, beyond recognition or gratification?"

Ironically, these jobs that we would gladly do for free are the ones where we could probably make the most money! When we put passion into our work, our customers and clients gladly seek our services. Think about it: How would you feel if you could have fun during your work day? How would that affect your eating habits?

AFFIRMATIONS FOR NUT CRAVERS

- It's okay to be good to myself.
- I follow my heart where it leads me.
- I realize that fun is a necessity.
- I enjoy myself; allowing time for pleasure and carefree activities.
- I love to let go and let my inner child experience unrestrained joy and freedom.
- I am responsible for meeting my needs; I give myself permission to have fun during the day.
- It's a sign of strength to take care of my aspirations and desires.

BREADS, RICE, AND PASTA:
COMFORTING AND CALMING

A hh...bread. Who can resist a steaming basket of freshly baked bread when it's placed in front of you in a restaurant? There are some aromas that bypass all defenses and logic, the smell of fresh-out-of-the-oven bread being one of them. You pull off a slice of the hot, sweet, and soft bread with its crispy crust, bite into it, and feel as if you're enveloped in a wave of euphoria.

The smell, the texture, the taste, and the inherent mood-altering properties of bread, rice, and pasta make them some of the foods that are most craved by stressed, tense, or frightened folks. The underlying FATS feelings with respect to starch cravings are Fear and Tension. Take Monica's case, for example.

A 42-year-old sales manager, Monica felt insecure about her job. She was at my stress-management workshop because she had just heard through the company grapevine that five management positions were being eliminated. Monica went 'round and 'round in her head, wondering if she would get a pink slip or not. For three months, Monica had endured this uncertainty. She was tense from not knowing what the future held for her, and not knowing whether she could count on drawing a steady income or not. Monica turned to bread to calm her weary nerves. Indulging in bread's soft texture was tantamount to a good friend putting a strong arm around her and saying, "Everything's going to be okay."

Many of the carbohydrate cravers I have worked with were experiencing high levels of life stress, and there is quite a bit of research showing that this is no coincidence. Researcher Sarah Leibowitz of Rockefeller University discovered that cortisol—the brain-produced hormone that anesthetizes pain—explains the tension/carbohydrate link. Here's how it works:

— When we get tense, our body assumes we are in danger and may need pain medication.
— The brain produces excess cortisol to anesthetize any pain.
— Cortisol, in turn, stimulates production of another brain chemical called "Neuropeptide Y." This chemical is a chief factor in turning carbohydrate cravings on and off.[1]
— The excess neuropeptide Y triggers carbohydrate cravings.
— If we eat in response to these cravings, we're more apt to gain weight. Neuropeptide Y and cortisol, still believing that the body may be in danger, order the body to hang on to any excess body fat.

Tension not only creates constant carbohydrate cravings, it also makes it more difficult to lose body fat!

Baking Bread and Lullabies

The smell of freshly baked bread reminds us of being in Mom's kitchen, where she is taking loving care of all our needs. She's tucking us in and reading us a bedtime story. We momentarily return to our early years, when things seemed a lot simpler and there weren't a lot of responsibilities.

Bread's sweet aroma fills our heart with the giddy lightness of a child on a swing. In fact, a survey of 1,000 people concluded that the smell of baked goods was the aroma that most reminded them of childhood.[2]

When life starts to feel brutal and uncaring, we crave a return to Mommy's nurturing arms. Bread cravings, especially for soft bread products, reflect our body's need for more tender loving care. Our peace of mind is out of balance because we feel misunderstood and unloved, as was the case with my client, Rebecca.

> Having just moved to a big city for a new job that she described as being filled with harsh office politics, Rebecca would go home at night alone and console herself with bread binges. It seemed that she had an insatiable appetite for soft rolls and biscuits.
>
> Rebecca's isolative habits were certainly understandable, but I refused to conspire with Rebecca in her belief that "It's poor li'l me against the harsh, bitter world." In the long run, that type of kindness would have been cruel on my part.
>
> Instead, we worked on *attracting* positive relationships into Rebecca's life. She went on the Negativity Diet described earlier, which helped her adopt a softer, friendlier demeanor. As she shed her belief that other people were out to get her, Rebecca's body language changed. She replaced defensiveness with an approachable air that said, "I'm your friend." Rebecca stood straight and wore a big smile. Her positive energy was contagious, and she told me, "I can't believe how much nicer everyone is to me. They've really changed!"
>
> As Rebecca felt safer and more loved, she lost her desire to binge on bread. She didn't *need* the craving anymore, because she was comfortable with her life and herself.

CARBOHYDRATE CRAVING SURVIVAL TIPS

✦ *Eat small snacks of carbohydrates*. By doing so, your carbohydrate cravings at the next meal will likely be reduced, according to research by Judith and Richard Wurtman. Try rice cakes or a bagel for your next snack, and see if your appetite for high-fat carbs is lessened at dinnertime.

✦ *Exercise.* One reason we crave carbohydrates is that we have low levels of the brain chemical, serotonin. Many studies show that even one session of exercise increases serotonin levels in the brain, and this effect will last throughout the day.[3] Even better, consistent exercise (defined as 30 minutes of aerobic activity six times a week) is one of the best ways to pump up your serotonin and tone down your carbohydrate cravings. In one study, consistent exercisers were found to have high amounts of serotonin that stayed at that level for up to seven days.[4] Exercise is slimming in more ways than one when it reduces your out-of-control cravings.

✦ *Take Vitamin B-6 supplements.* This, too, will keep your serotonin levels high enough to combat carbohydrate cravings. About 100 mg of B-6 per day is considered an optimum dosage for serotonin maintenance, and is considered a safe dosage by many experts (although you may want to check with your doctor first).[5]

✦ *Choose low-fat carbohydrates.* Joseph Piscatella, author of *Controlling Your Fat Tooth,* knows the importance of this advice from personal experience. At age 32, Piscatella underwent open-heart coronary bypass surgery—a wake-up call alerting him to the life-or-death consequences of not eating right. Today, he counsels and writes about choosing low-fat carbohydrate snacks, including air-popped popcorn (no butter), rice

cakes, corn tortillas, cereals, and bread sticks for crunchy cravings. For sweet, smooth cravings, Piscatella recommends angel
food cake, tapioca, and gelatin.[6]

✦ *Take any steps you can to de-stress your life.* Okay, so you'd
love to quit your job and move to a tropical island! Still,
there are more practical and much less radical ways to reduce
stress. After all, stress and tension lead to the comfort cravings
underneath an out-of-control appetite for carbohydrates.
And since stress also depletes serotonin, stressed-out carbohydrate cravers become trapped in a frightening cycle of
stress-eat/stress-eat.

Ask yourself, "What one step can I take right now that will
afford me some relief from my stress?" This may involve:

— *Writing down your priorities* and eliminating nonessential activities from your schedule. If a time-consuming
activity is not contributing to your health or happiness
or to that of your family or your favorite cause, then
why bother?

— *Asking your family to help you.* Any child over the age
of three can help with household chores. Children also
feel important when you give them little jobs. And
don't forget to assign Daddy some tasks, too!

— *Working smarter at your job.* An eye-opening study by
the research firm Robert Half & Associates has shown
that four hours a day are wasted at work on needless
socializing. This means that the average employee only
spends four hours focused on work. Many people feel
stressed when they leave the office because they feel
burdened by unfinished projects. If you can eliminate
even half of the extraneous socializing that erodes your

productive time at your job, you'll arrive home feeling more satisfied and settled.

✦ ***Seek out nonfood means of comfort.*** Some of my clients use teddy bears as a substitute for food when they are embarking on their recovery from food cravings. They hug the bear instead of opening the cupboard. Other people turn to pets for comfort as a substitute for binge-eating on bread. Even better: seek out human comfort. A close, warm, and emotionally vulnerable relationship with another person is the most effective source of comfort available. Here's a good affirmation for healing relationship problems: *"My life is in harmony, and my heart is filled with love and laughter. I am a good friend and am rewarded with nurturing friendships. I attract loving people and am surrounded by warmth and love right now."*

AFFIRMATIONS FOR CARBOHYDRATE CRAVERS

ે Anything I lose will automatically be replaced with something better.

ે I am relaxed and trusting, right now.

ે I release my tension into the universe.

ે Love is surrounding me right at this very moment.

ે My source of love is within me and around me at all times.

ે I have enough time, talent, and energy to accomplish all my goals.

ે My friends are loving people who reach out to comfort me.

ે   ે   ે

COOKIES, CAKES, AND PIES: CRAVING HUGS, PLEASURE, AND REASSURANCE

S weet carbohydrate cravings are similar to those for bread, rice, and pasta. Both food groups are high in carbohydrates, which produce soothing emotions. Their chewy, soft texture functions as an edible hug. Yet, sweet carbohydrate cravings—for cookie dough, cookies, cakes, and pies—represent another element that sets this food category apart from unsweetened bread. They correspond to a desire for comfort and reassurance, as bread does, but they can also signal resistance to doing something (procrastination), and relate to feelings similar to those that a hurt child has who needs a hug from Mommy. My client Leticia is a prime example:

— Leticia had promised herself that she'd clean out the garage this weekend, but here it was, Saturday afternoon, and she wasn't even close to starting the project. Instead, she was in the kitchen, hypnotically eating soft chocolate chip cookies. One after another. Leticia's cookie cravings were her way of fending off thoughts such as, "My husband should be the one cleaning the garage—not me!"

— Another client, Corinne, was procrastinating with respect to an even more emotionally volatile act: filing for divorce. She had caught her husband cheating and couldn't reconcile her feelings of betrayal. Corinne knew, in her heart, that her marriage could never be the same. She had the divorce attorney's telephone number in front of her. Yet, every time she'd pick up the phone to make an appointment, she'd feel overwhelming cravings for chocolate cake. Corinne needed reassurance that filing for divorce was the best choice.

When Food Is Love

Some preferences for sweets are learned, because we were often rewarded for good behavior in childhood with a candy treat. Two studies by noted nutritional researcher and author, L.L. Birch, underscore the power of this sweets-as-reward experience.

In one study, the researcher tried to bribe children to eat a disliked food such as spinach or liver. The children were told, "If you eat that food, you'll get a cookie as a reward." The bribe didn't produce the desired results, because the children's appetite for the disliked food actually decreased. The more they were bribed with the promise of a sweet reward, the less the children preferred the taste of the vegetables or meats.

In Birch's second study, children were offered food as a reward for performing some chore. For example, if a child cleaned the chalkboard, she was given a cookie. If she performed a math problem correctly, she got to eat some cake. All of the food rewards consisted of those that the children already liked prior to the experiment.

But here's the surprising result: the children's preferences for these cakes and cookies markedly increased after the foods were used as rewards! Somehow, the foods' "value" increased for the children. Now, these foods were no longer just delicious, but they were viewed as a commodity and as a reward.[1]

Most likely, these two study results are a function of the "extrinsic reward" phenomenon. If we are paid or bribed to engage in an activity—even one that we would normally choose to do for free—we enjoy that activity less. We move from an "intrinsic reward" position, of doing the behavior because we enjoy it to an "extrinsic reward" position, or performing the behavior to acquire an outside reward.

This phenomenon explains why, if you've ever tried to turn your favorite hobby into a salaried job, you'll find that your enjoyment drops a couple of notches. I remember this happening to me when I held a part-time job reviewing feature movies for a local television station. I love going to the movies, but because I suddenly *had* to watch films it was no longer the pleasant pastime I'd once enjoyed (and I found that I also developed an aversion to popcorn!).

With extrinsic rewards, you're no longer engaged in the activity because you choose to. You're doing it because you're being paid to do it—although this sort of job usually beats all the other types of jobs, hands down!

If you're a parent, then this study provides valuable information. We can't bribe our kids with cookies to eat their vegetables! Not only will they learn to dislike vegetables, but they'll also learn to like cookies so much that they may develop a Constant Craving.

If you experience overwhelming cravings for cookies, cakes, or pie, you may want to think back to childhood experiences where you may have been rewarded with these foods. This is not an attempt to blame the adults in your life. Instead, it's a means of trying to understand your cravings in order to reduce or eliminate them.

Ask yourself:

+ Do I remember my parents, teachers, or babysitters bribing me with sweet treats in order to get me to finish my chores or homework?
+ Did anyone give me cake because I was being a good little child?
+ Did my neighbors reward me with cookies because I was helpful?

✦ Did someone give me sweets to pacify me when I was crying or upset?

✦ When I'd go shopping with my mother, would she invariably stop at the bakery to get me a cookie?

✦ Did I learn to associate birthdays, holidays, and other special occasions with cake, cookies, and pie?

✦ Did I feel loved whenever someone would bake me a cake or some cookies?

✦ Do I associate the smell of baking cookies with feelings of love and pleasure?

✦ Do I reward my own children or other loved ones by baking or buying them cookies or cakes?

WAYS TO COMBAT COOKIE, CAKE, AND PIE CRAVINGS

✦ *Heal the self-esteem.* Self-Esteem Eaters (see Chapter 4) are especially prone to cookie cravings. Usually, there are unresolved issues from childhood that are calling out for your acknowledgment and attention. What messages in your childhood did you learn that are affecting your self-esteem today? As an adult, you can heal your self-esteem by consistently treating yourself in self-loving ways, such as:

— *Guarding against negativity* (see the Negativity Diet in Chapter 10). Avoid any negative self-talk. Your unconscious believes every word you say about yourself, whether you intend it as a joke or not. Do not allow other people to put you down in their words or their actions. Immediately tell the other person what you will and won't accept in your relationship.

— *Taking excellent care of your body.* Exercise, eat a balanced diet, and maintain regular sleep habits.

— *Giving yourself lots of hugs.* Acknowledge your successes to yourself. Give yourself a compliment. Write yourself a love letter. Develop ways to become your own best friend.

✦ ***Reward yourself with nonfood treats.*** As we've seen in this chapter, some of our cookie cravings stem from the childhood message that "sweets equal rewards." We all need pats on the back and kudos for hard work. But instead of stopping at the cookie shop for your reward, why not instead treat yourself to a new C.D., a book, an item of clothing, scented soap, theater tickets, or a piece of jewelry? They are less fattening and infinitely more satisfying than a cookie!

✦ ***Watch out for black-and-white thinking.*** Lorraine would always open the bag of Oreo cookies with the best intentions of just eating one. But there was something about the sight of that unfinished row of cookies that really bugged her. So she'd eat *all* the cookies in the row. This act gave her a sense of relief and completion. Behavioral scientists call this mental habit "black-and-white thinking." It reflects an uncompromising desire to complete something, whether it is healthy or not. This all-or-nothing thought process also correlates to obsessive-compulsiveness and many types of addictions.

AFFIRMATIONS FOR COOKIE, CAKE, AND PIE CRAVINGS

- I am loved, and I am lovable.

- I am a good person, and other people naturally like who I am.

- It's okay to give myself hugs and appreciation.

- When I win, others win.

- I am now enveloped in warm, delicious love.

- If it's going to be, it's up to me!

CANDY CRAVINGS:
SWEET PICK-ME-UPS, REWARDS,
AND ENTERTAINMENT

A woman named Karen who attended one of my seminars told me that she couldn't relate to chocoholics. She loved candy but could not understand why anyone would choose a chocolate kiss over a lemon drop. Karen adored hard candies.

She regularly bought bags of hard candies, in different flavors, when she went grocery shopping. Some of the candy went to her young son, Mark, and sometimes her husband got to eat a delicious fruit candy or a jelly bean. But most of it was reserved especially for Karen.

Karen had a comfortable life—nothing much to complain about. She held a part-time job as the secretary of her church, and her husband was the manager of a manufacturing plant, a job he'd held for 25 years. They also had two cars and a well-behaved son. So why was Karen overeating hard candies? After all, her life was seemingly stable and free of any stress.

Well, a study by a leading nutritional researcher may explain Karen's cravings. This study compared 40 candy cravers with 40 people who didn't care for candy. No differences were found as far as the amount of calories, carbohydrates, protein, or fat that the two groups normally consumed.

There was only one difference between the two groups: Candy cravers reported more boredom and less stress than the group not craving candy. Furthermore, the candy cravers displayed high levels of guilt for their cravings—that is, whenever they'd succumb to a candy-eating binge, they'd feel guilty. The Candy Bingers would think, "Well, I've blown my diet. I may as well eat whatever I like and start my diet again tomorrow."[1]

Cravings for sweets, as I've stated before, appear to be innate. From the 1920s to the 1930s, a famous study of infants showed the degree of humans' incredible preferences for sweets. The infants were given any food that they pointed to, and the vast majority of children pointed to the sweetest foods available—fruit.[2]

We've held a cultural belief for ages that sugar causes hyperactivity, especially in children. To test the validity of this belief, research scientist Judith Rapoport placed a newspaper advertisement specifically recruiting children who, after eating sugar, were more active.

Many mothers agreed to let their children participate in the study, claiming that their offspring became hyperactive in response to even minute tastes of sugar. The study divided these children into two groups—those who received sugar and those who didn't. The before-and-after sugar-activity levels of both groups would be compared for differences. Rapoport conducted a double-blind experiment, so she wouldn't know which children were receiving sugar, and which were receiving a sugar-free substitute. She didn't want to risk influencing the outcome of the study.

The results were surprising! The children receiving sugar did not become more active. In fact, they showed signs of lethargy and decreased activity after eating the sugar.[3] The results may have come from increased serotonin from the sugar's carbohydrate structure, which was responsible for the lethargy. Serotonin, of course, regulates mood and energy. When serotonin levels are high, we feel calm or even sleepy. Other theories about the "crash" following a sugar high hinge on blood-sugar fluctuations.[4]

Yet, due to the widespread belief that sugar acts as a pick-me-up, many of us turn to a candy bar when our energy levels begin to dip. The biological result is an up-and-down energy fluctuation. We eat more candy to get that initial boost once again.

Sweets—the Earliest Craving

Several researchers have studied the innate desire for sweets in human infants. Newborn infants were presented with a choice of sweetened fluid and plain water. Which liquid do you suppose the babies preferred? Even one-day-old infants drank more when given sweet fluids. Not only that, but the sweeter the concentration of fluids, the more liquid the babies consumed.[5] Many researchers conclude, from studies such as this, that we have an innate preference for sweets.

Our human appetite for sweets may have arisen in our ancient primate ancestors. Monkeys and other primates show a preference for sweet fruits over any other type of food. Some researchers speculate that fruits were a sure source of calories and energy for our cave-dwelling ancestors, and we developed a natural affinity for sweet stuff as a result of survival instincts. Along the same lines, we "knew" that sweetness equated ripeness when we were foraging for food in the wild. (All animals, in fact, prefer sweets over other types of foods. Studies with horses, bears, and ants show a universal love for sugary-sweet foods.)

I, too, believe that we have inherited our "sweet tooth" from our ancestors (both animal and human) who knew how to scavenge for a tree-ripened piece of fruit. Their instinctive wisdom told them to seek out the sweetest of fruits, since sweetness signals a safe food that is ripe and full of vitamins and energy-producing calories. Our instincts to seek out sweet-tasting fruit have been bastardized today, twisted into an appetite for candies.

One reason for our "modern" cravings is the lack of truly sweet fruit at most grocery stores. We have a vast array of produce available to us, but most of the selection is artificially ripened, taste-less, and not sufficiently sweet to satisfy us.

WAYS TO COMBAT SWEET CRAVINGS

+ *Buy fruit at a reliable fruit stand.* If you ask around, your co-workers or neighbors will probably be able to tell you the name of a hole-in-the-wall fruit stand that sells delicious fruit. Usually, these fruit stands buy directly from local growers and sell tree-ripened fruit. It makes a big difference, so it is worth driving out of your way.

+ *Keep fruit handy.* If you're stressed, you don't want to hassle with any difficult-to-prepare foods. You want something quick, easy-to-fix, and delicious. You'll do yourself a favor by anticipating this normal human desire. Preslice your fruit, squeeze a little lemon juice over it to prevent browning, cover it with clear plastic (so you'll see it), and keep it on an ac-cessible refrigerator shelf. Keep washed grapes in a big bowl. Place bananas within eyesight. The more available your fresh fruit is, the more apt you are to eat it.

+ *Make fruit a special treat.* One reason we shun fruit during our sweet cravings is that fruit seems like a deprivation alternative. We've got to dress fruit up! Put a little flavored, fat-free yo-gurt on top of your fruit (and maybe a mint sprig, too!) and you've got a gourmet dessert. Purée fruit with an ice cube and some ginger ale, and you've got a sorbet. Microwave sliced apples for two minutes at high temperature, top with cinna-mon, and you've got a quick, low-calorie apple pie-type treat.

+ *Try frozen fruit.* When fresh fruit becomes scarce during the winter, a good alternative awaits you in the freezer aisle. Have you ever tried fruits that are frozen in one-pound plastic bags?

They cost a little more than fresh fruit, and they are a little mushy when thawed, but they are extremely sweet and flavorful, even though they are unsweetened. I like thawed frozen fruit as a breakfast accompaniment to cereal, cottage cheese, or yogurt.

✦ *Avoid the tendency to overeat fat-free sweets.* Several cookie companies are making fortunes off the current fat-free fad. We all want to have our cake and eat it, too. But we can't consume a whole box of fudge cookies—at 50 calories per cookie—and expect to lose or even maintain our weight. That's magical thinking, a product of the cookie company's clever marketing.

✦ *Analyze your candy cravings.*

— Are you craving red-hot candies? That's a signal that you are craving more excitement.
— Are you craving cinnamon hard candies? That's a sign that you are feeling tense and frightened. Cinnamon warms the body and reduces blood pressure. Interestingly enough, cinnamon has been the base ingredient in Chinese herbal medicine for hundreds of years.[6]
— Are you craving peppermints? That means you're feeling lethargic and want to catch your second breath of peppy energy.
— Are you craving coffee candy? That means you are trying to push yourself past the point of exhaustion. Why not take a breather (or better yet, a nap)?
— Are you craving peanut brittle? This signals a frustration that your life lacks fun or recreation. You're also looking for a little sympathy or comfort.
— Are you craving caramel? You may be struggling with some indecision. It's probably creating internal stress because you don't know which choices to make.

— Is your craving for licorice? Licorice, like cinnamon, has been a basic Chinese remedy for many years. It has been prescribed for anxiety and stress, especially in women. Licorice is seen as a cure-all for tension, one which will increase energy.[7] Since chewy foods alleviate stress, perhaps part of the effectiveness lies in licorice's chewy texture.

— Are you craving jelly beans? That can mean you're juggling an abundance of responsibilities, being forced to make too many important decisions in rapid-fire succession. This situation may be creating some anxiety in you, but not that much; after all, you're still full of confidence.

— Are you craving a hard candy that you can bite your teeth into? That desire to crunch indicates some internal stress, anger, or anxiety.

— Are you craving a sucker, or some other candy that you can suck on? This signifies some boredom or impatience, a "Come on, let's get this show on the road" frustration. But because you don't have complete control over the situation, you're relegated to sitting back and waiting—a situation you don't enjoy, nor do you agree with.

✦ *Directly confront the underlying emotional issues.* If, after analyzing your cravings, you discover any anger, stress, or frustration, ask yourself how you might take even one step toward alleviating the source of those emotions. Is there someone you can talk to, or some changes you can make in your life? If you reduce the source of your uncomfortable emotions, you won't need to crave sweets anymore.

✦ *Avoid keeping sweets readily available or highly visible.* Studies show that certain types of people are more prone to emotional overeating than others. These include obese people and those who are more focused on others than they are on themselves. These two "types" are more apt to eat in response to stress or emotional upset, especially if some delicious food is right there for the taking.

Make it difficult to binge-eat on candy by removing it from your home, your car, or your office space. Having a candy jar on your desk is not a good idea if you're a Sweets Craver. Keeping candy on your coffee table for guests to nibble on is not a good idea either. Remember, your kids and husband don't need candy in the house! Most of the Sweets Cravers I've worked with buy candy for themselves, but rationalize that, "It's for my family." In reality, the family eats one or two pieces, and the Sweets Craver eats 25 pieces. A major step in recovering from overwhelming food cravings is developing self-honesty about one's motives for buying food. Don't wait to give the candy to your neighbor—that's another rationalization! Get rid of it right now. Destroy it.

✦ ***Allow yourself moderate portions of candy.*** I'm not advocating total abstinence from candy; far from it. In fact, I think eating binges are often products of excessive deprivation. I used to do that very thing myself. I'd swear off of candy and sweets, but deep down would feel sorry for myself for being so deprived. I felt like a little girl whose mother brought all her siblings a candy, but didn't give any to her. I'd go for two or three months completely abstaining from all sugared products. Then, I'd get fed up and go to the other extreme. I'd buy giant-size candy bars and eagerly take them home and indulge in a secret binge-eating session. Was I overcompensating for all those days and weeks away from candy? Yes, you better believe it! That's why I believe in moderation. Instead of seesawing between the two extremes of either bringing home huge bags of candy or completely abstaining, here are some realistic alternatives:

— *Buy candy in one-serving portions.* Most supermarkets sell candy in bulk. Pick out just the amount of candy you plan to eat at one time, and then put one-half that amount back on the shelf. In this way, you'll fulfill your candy cravings but won't overdo it.

— *Be aware of all-or-nothing thinking.* According to Jane Hirschmann and Carol Munter, authors of *When Women Stop Hating Their Bodies*, when we tell ourselves, "This is the last time I'll ever be able to eat candy; I'd better eat enough to satisfy me because I'll never get this chance again," we create so much anxiety within ourselves that it's almost a certainty that we'll go on an eating binge. It's like we're seeing a beloved person for the last time, so of course we want to spend as much time as possible with that object of our affection.[7]

AFFIRMATIONS FOR SWEET CRAVINGS

- Time is an unlimited resource.
- I have enough energy to accomplish all my goals.
- I live my life in accordance with my inner voice.
- I trust my intuition to guide and direct me.
- It's okay for me to seek recreation and entertainment.

HIGH-FAT FOODS:
FILLING THE EMPTINESS

The fat content in the food we crave has quite a bit of significance. While studies show that most people prefer high-fat foods when they feel calorie deprived (such as during the typical diet), there are people who have overwhelming cravings for high-fat foods. These are folks who practically live at fast-food restaurants, where greasy cheeseburgers and oily french fries are a staple of daily life.

High-fat diets indicate a fear of feeling empty. Fatty foods stay in the stomach much longer than low-fat foods, which digest and pass through the system rather rapidly. High-Fat Cravers are afraid of facing the prospect of an empty stomach, so they ensure that their bellies are full by continually tanking up on high-fat foods.

Often, the High-Fat Eater is deeply afraid of something. Of being alone. Of facing a terrible truth. Of taking responsibility. Of making changes. These fears and insecurities are quelled by a consistently plugged stomach.

High-fat food cravings include those for cheeseburgers, soft french fries, or onion rings and soft fried foods. Fatty versions of meat, such as soft-fried chicken, marbled steak, fatty prime rib, ham, and pork also fall into this category.

The emptiness that High-Fat Eaters fear often stems from a lack of meaning or purpose in their lives. Often, the High-Fat Eater is a person who would like to change careers or return to school but fears failure or change. Fat fills up the stomach and blocks the awareness of emptiness pangs. But as soon as the stomach empties, the person's cravings for high-fat food returns.

High-fat cravers often live painful lives. They sometimes set themselves up so that other people will hurt them, either emotionally or physically. They hurt and betray themselves. And often, they don't know that they have the right to insist that this mistreatment should stop. They are also afraid to speak up and say, "No! You're hurting me!" Pamela is a good example:

An attendee at one of my seminars, Pamela stated that she believed that all men would always betray her and cheat on her. She had been in a three-year relationship with Marcus, a man who wanted to marry her. But Pamela was sure that Marcus would leave her for another woman, always thinking, "I'm too fat to keep a man's attention for long."

Every time Marcus would suggest marriage, Pamela would decline or change the subject. Although, as Pamela described him, Marcus was a loving man, everyone has their limits; healthy people don't hang on to unhealthy relationships. When he finally figured out that Pamela wasn't capable of giving or receiving love, he broke up with her.

So, Pamela's worst fears were confirmed, but only because she'd made them come true. Before she came to my seminar, she went on a high-fat eating binge that lasted three weeks. "I want to get into another relationship, but I'm afraid of being betrayed again," she bemoaned. I pointed out to Pamela that she had, in fact, betrayed herself by pushing Marcus away. She agreed, saying that this insight instilled her with hope. "I won't repeat the same mistake twice," she told me and the seminar audience. I hope she means it.

Fat-Foraging: A Survival Skill?

Fat cravings appear to be one of our innate drives. Experiments with rats, as well as with humans, show how nature has equipped us with a preference for high-fat foods.

Rats, in one study, were offered two types of foods with very distinct flavors. The two foods were also different in that one was high-fat, and the other food was low-fat. Let's call the high-fat food "Flavor A" and the low-fat food "Flavor B." The rats learned to associate Flavor A with high-fat content.

Next, the researchers presented the rats with two foods with identical fat content, and with the two different types of Flavors, A and B. All the rats preferred the Flavor A foods, even though it now had the same fat content as Flavor B. The rats had learned to associate that flavor with a high-fat content![1]

Fat-paired-with-flavor conditioned response experiments have also been conducted on humans, with similar results. One study tested adult subjects, and the other study used preschool children. In both, the researchers gave the subjects a high-fat food with a strong and distinctive flavor, such as barbecue or teriyaki. Soon, the subjects learned to pair this flavor with a high-fat content. And since a high fat-content leads to greater and quicker feelings of fullness, the subjects associated the flavor with "feeling full."

Next, the researchers gave subjects a low-fat food flavored in the same way as the high-fat food. Even though the subjects were now consuming a low-fat meal, they responded as if the food was still high-fat. The conditioning of the flavor resulted in subjects reporting feeling full much sooner than when they ate a similar meal not containing the flavor.[2]

Through analysis of these studies, researcher A.W. Logue concluded:

> Fat is much denser in calories than are proteins or carbohydrates (fat contains 9 calories per gram, but proteins and

carbohydrates each contain 4 calories per gram). Perhaps humans learn to like relatively high-calorie foods, including foods that are high in fat, because of their caloric consequences.

It is not surprising that humans and other animals are able to learn which foods are dense in calories and that they prefer those foods. Such behavior would be adaptive for species such as ours that evolved in food-scarce environments. Unfortunately, now that food is no longer scarce for most people in the United States, our preferences for high-calorie food make it difficult to keep fat consumption low....[3]

Overcoming Fat Cravings

Fat Cravers endure an especially painful struggle, because they compound their feelings of emptiness by eating foods virtually guaranteed to add pounds to their body. With the added weight comes a degree of social ostracism and prejudice, including job discrimination, negative feedback from romantic partners, and feeling like an invisible member of society. These signals that overweight people somehow aren't as valuable as thin people, hurt. They make the Fat Craver feel even more alone and empty, which, in turn, trigger still more Fat Cravings.

To break this cycle, Fat Cravers need more courage than any other Constant Craver. The emptiness inside of Fat Cravers makes it difficult for them to trust other people's advice, even when they know that a great deal of wisdom may be imparted to them. So, I am going to ask you, the Fat Craver, to suspend disbelief and mistrust momentarily and give these suggestions a try. You will always be in control every moment, and you can always stop at any time.

ADVICE FOR FAT CRAVERS

✦ *Fill your heart with substance.* Distract yourself from your thoughts about food by keeping busy with soul-nourishing activities. These could include attending a spiritual study group, the theater, concerts, joining a choir, or forming a group your-self related to one of your interests.

✦ ***Exercise.*** As is the case with other types of cravings, studies show that exercise reduces the appetite for dietary fat signif-icantly. This is especially true for yo-yo dieters, whose weight has gone up and down. People in this category have the strongest fat cravings of virtually any group. Yo-Yo Syndrome sufferers also display the most dramatic decreases in fat crav-ings in response to exercise.

✦ ***Work on the issues triggering feelings of emptiness.*** Often, empty pangs stem from unexamined childhood issues. Is there something from your childhood that you want to confront? Some painful anger or guilt you are holding onto that needs brief examination? After you confront the issue, either through honest introspection or by talking with a trusted psy-chotherapist, be sure to release it from your body and mind.

Are you stuck, wondering what childhood issues might possi-bly be triggering your empty feelings? One clue is the place on your body where fat is carried. I learned from Louise Hay's in-terpretations in her wonderful book, *Heal Your Body*, that fat stored in the thighs, for example, stems from "packed childhood anger. Often rage at the father." Louise suggests this affirmation as an antidote: *"I see my father as a loveless child and I forgive easily. We are both free."*[4]

Louise also states that belly fat signifies "anger at being denied nourishment." This coincides with my findings that fat around the stomach is related to anger towards one's mother.

It's difficult to admit feeling anger toward a parent. The resid-ual childhood belief is that our parents will abandon us if we ex-press anger toward them. And abandonment would feel worse than anything we feel now. We're always so afraid of making things worse! Usually, that is an unsubstantiated fear that is covering up our true fear that we aren't strong enough to be authentic and honest. Yet, that is our real source of strength.

If you are carrying weight on your thighs, ask yourself, "Could I possibly be carrying around resentment toward my father?" If the answer is yes, ask yourself, "What steps can I take right now to release this pain?"

If you are carrying around stomach weight, ask yourself, "Could I possibly be carrying around resentment toward my mother?" If that answer is yes, ask yourself, "What steps can I take right now to release this pain?"

Emotional or physical pain is always a sign that something is amiss. This type of pain is not meant to be blindly accepted; instead it is a messenger demanding our attention. In my book, *Losing Your Pounds of Pain: Breaking the Link Between Abuse, Stress, and Overeating*, I go into great detail about ways to deal with childhood pain resulting from physical, sexual, and emotional abuse. I urge you to seek these healthier alternatives as a means of releasing yourself from the bondage of resentment.

AFFIRMATIONS FOR HIGH-FAT CRAVINGS

🐾 I have the power and intelligence to make decisions.

🐾 I am loved and secure, and I feel these emotions from deep within myself.

🐾 God's love lives within me, through and through.

🐾 It's okay for me to be alone.

🐾 All my needs are taken care of right now.

🐾 I am safe; I am bathed in warm, white light.

🐾 I am responsible for myself, and I make sure other people are aware of my boundaries.

🐾 🐾 🐾

LOVE IS THE FILLING FEELING

Throughout this book, I have emphasized the underlying emotional, spiritual, and psychological reasons behind food cravings. Scientific research cited in this book confirms the link between people's moods and their corresponding food cravings. It also reveals the correlation between the spirit and the body.

We are spiritual beings who inhabit a body that is perfect, whole, and complete. Every part of our body responds to our beliefs, thoughts, and emotions. When one part of the body appears to be malfunctioning, we must look at the thought that needs healing. Heal the thought and we heal the body.

A negative and a positive emotion cannot simultaneously occupy the same space. You either feel fear or you feel love. If you are living in Fear, or its manifestations of Anger, Tension, or Shame, the solution is to pour love on the situation. Fill yourself up with love, and the negative emotions have no place to live.

Our gut is the center of all emotions, negative and positive. We are guided by gut feelings, which tell us which path to take and which people to associate with. Sometimes, these gut feelings scare us because we believe we will fail to fulfill our dreams. And when we feel frightened, we try to drown out the voice of our gut feelings by pouring food on them.

So, you can pour one of two things on your gut feelings: food or love. Pouring food on your gut is easy; we all know how to do that. Pouring love on your gut requires some patience and practice, but it is worth it! Remember to always look for that little feeling of a butterfly in your stomach. Ask it to expand into a glorious feeling of love and childlike fun. This feeling is filling, and the gut is so stuffed with love that Fear, Anger, Tension, and Shame are evicted from your body like unwanted tenants.

Paying attention to your gut feelings means that you trust that you have the talent, time, energy, money, intelligence, and creativity to fulfill your dreams. This trust comes from a faith that you were born in the image and likeness of your Creator. When you follow your gut, you are rewarded with a satisfying existence.

When we ignore our gut, our FATS feelings of Fear, Anger, Tension, and Shame grow louder and larger. These feelings rob us of our inner harmony.

Here is the important bottom line: we crave foods and overeat in an attempt to regain equilibrium and peace of mind. Our cravings are always for foods that correspond to our ignored gut feeling. If your gut is telling you to have more fun, but you ignore your gut, you will crave a food that contains pyrozine, such as peanut butter, cashews, or walnuts. That is because pyrozine triggers the pleasure center of your brain. The body always attempts to achieve homeostasis, and if you ignore your gut feelings, your appetite will seek to fulfill the body's needs through food cravings.

The most direct method to reduce or eliminate your Constant Craving is to listen to, trust, and then follow your gut feelings. You will know when the message comes from your gut, and not from your human will, by setting aside daily quiet time for meditation, prayer, or affirmations. A true gut feeling will always be born in love, and will be an activity that meshes with your natural talents and interests. Your gut will always direct you toward activities that benefit other people, and never toward those that involve dishonor or deception.

When you get into the healthy habit of following your gut, you will always be rewarded with remarkable experiences. One of the miracles you'll enjoy is a normal appetite, and a naturally low body weight.

We are meant to have a free spirit and a light body. Everybody has a Divine right to love, fun, creative expression, perfect health, and prosperity. When you claim your rights, your body responds in gratitude and harmony. Suddenly, you are no longer fighting your appetite.

When your appetite normalizes, your excess body weight will drop off naturally, almost without thought. Then, as long as you maintain your peace of mind, you will not struggle with food cravings. *Long-term weight maintenance, then, is actually peace-of-mind maintenance.*

It takes practice and vigilance to stay centered in a peace-of-mind framework, though. It's sometimes difficult to stay in a state of tranquil bliss. And that's where food cravings are your best ally. As soon as a craving comes up, analyze it and pinpoint the issue in your gut feelings that needs addressing. Voilà! Back to peace of mind, as well as a normal appetite!

ॐ   ॐ   ॐ

THE
CRAVINGS
CHART

CHARTING YOUR FOOD CRAVINGS

W hat follows is a chart of foods that are commonly craved. It was inspired by Louise Hay's uniquely helpful lists of physical ailments, their corresponding mental thought patterns, and her suggested healing affirmations in her books *Heal Your Body* and *You Can Heal Your Life*.[1] This chart will help you uncover the underlying feelings triggering your particular Constant Craving.

One reminder is that this chart refers to food *cravings*, not food preferences. A craving is a persistent and overwhelming desire to eat a particular food. Emotional hunger is intense, sudden hunger that appears in your mind and your mouth. Physical hunger, on the other hand, is a gradual process that occurs in the stomach. A craving is also different from wanting a piece of cake or a cookie simply because you happen to see or smell that food. A food craving doesn't originate from contact with the food. Rather, the idea and flavor of the food enters our mind, triggering urges to seek out that food and overeat. They are Constant Cravings, only alleviated by directly addressing the underlying emotional cause.

Each craving is triggered by one or more of the FATS Feelings: Fear or its manifestations of Anger, Tension, and Shame. Those are the core emotions that inspire cravings for each particular food.

When we ignore our gut feelings and inner voice, we lose peace of mind. The body attempts to correct this imbalance and return itself to a state of homeostasis, or a state of balanced harmony. If we resist the gut's directions when confronting a troubling circumstance head-on, the body settles for a less satisfactory alternative. Your body knows that if you ingest a certain food, your emotions will be temporarily soothed. Your food cravings urge you to eat the food that matches your emotional circumstance. If you are depressed, you will feel hungry for an antidepressant food. If you are anxious, you will crave a calming food. Your cravings are signals that your body wants you to feel at peace.

Of course, eating food—just like taking antidepressant medication—doesn't fix the underlying problem. But sometimes we don't know how to go about fixing our circumstances. We're confused when it comes to decoding which voice is our inner guide and which voice is just our human desire to control outcomes. All we know is that we feel unsettled and hungry. When you interpret your food craving, you pinpoint which voice belongs to your inner guide.

This chart lists the probable meaning behind your food craving. If the description does not exactly pertain to your current circumstances, try asking yourself, "Am I feeling Fear, or its manifestations of Anger, Tension, or Shame right now?" When the true answer comes to you, it will "click." You will know what issue has diminished your peace of mind. Then, ask yourself what action you can take right this moment to begin correcting the troubling situation. Even one small step represents a decision to recover your calmness, your balance, your inner harmony. You will feel better when you make that decision, and your gut will no longer have to seek homeostasis through food cravings.

Affirmations for each food craving are also listed. The stronger and more persistent the craving, the more times you'll want to write and say each affirmation. If you have a negative thought after saying the affirmation, know that this negative thought comes from your Fear or its manifestations of Anger, Tension, or Shame. Know that only thoughts born of love are real. Negative thoughts are mental habits that can be healed by consistently affirming these self-loving thoughts for 30 days.

Food Craved	Probable Meaning	Affirmation
APPLE PIE, PLAIN	A desire for comfort, safety, and reassurance. Loneliness.	I am warmed by the love I feel inside me now.
APPLE PIE, WITH ICE CREAM / WHIPPED CREAM	Discouraged and depressed. Feeling like others don't care.	I trust with all my heart and know that good is coming to me now.
APPLESAUCE, PLAIN	Desiring energy and renewal.	I give myself permission to relax and let go.
APPLESAUCE WITH CINNAMON	Feeling alone and tense and desiring a fresh start. Self-blame: seeking relief and forgiveness.	I have love inside of me, which warms me and keeps me safe.
AVOCADO	Fed-up. Wanting to replace high-stress situation with something that better suits you.	I have decided to seek a better life, and am rewarded with answers and direction.
BACON (see "Pork")		
BAGEL (see "Bread")		

Food Craved	Probable Meaning	Affirmation
BATTER, CAKE (chocolate)	Fear of abandonment. Desiring love, hugs, and reassurance.	God's love is always with me, and I am never alone.
BATTER, CAKE (vanilla)	Insecure and feeling wounded. Feeling afraid and vulnerable to attack.	Love provides strength and wisdom in all my thoughts and actions.
BATTER, CHOCOLATE CHIP COOKIE	Insecure and feeling attacked by love partner. Also, angry at self.	It is safe to express my true feelings; I forgive and I love.
BATTER, PANCAKE	Desiring hugs, but afraid to accept love. Fear of rejection.	I accept the love that is within me; it warms me through and through.
BEEF		
Cheeseburger	Frightened by a sense of inner emptiness or inadequacy, and feeling depression. Fear of failure.	My source of strength and peace is within me right now. I let go of the belief that I am in control, and put my trust in my Creator.
Hamburger	Feeling insecure and unclear. Wanting direction, motivation, and energy.	I release my life to the universe, knowing that God has wonderful plans for me. When I follow these plans, all the details are taken care of.

Food Craved	Probable Meaning	Affirmation
Meat loaf	Desiring comfort, escape, and understanding. Feeling unsafe.	As I radiate love and shine my positive light on my life and others, all negative influences fall away naturally.
Pot pie	Anxiety, worry, and self-blame. Being too hard on self.	I deserve love just for being who I am now.
Steak	Tired because of stress. Wanting solutions and energy.	I have abundant time and energy. The universe has unlimited resources that flow through me now.
Stew	Feeling attacked and wanting understanding.	I am gentle and loving with myself. I manifest peace in my mind and my heart.
Stroganoff w/ beef and noodles or rice	Worry is leading to an energy drain and some self-blame. Wanting relief and energy.	I have the right to rest and relax. I take time to meet my needs.
BEER	Desire to shut out anxiety. Wanting more love, fun, and appreciation.	I trust my inner source of strength to see me through the highs and lows. I allow myself a quiet time-out for renewal.

BISCUITS (see "Bread")

Food Craved	Probable Meaning	Affirmation
BLUE CHEESE SALAD DRESSING (alone)	Feeling stuck or trapped. Depressed and wanting change, but afraid to take action.	It is safe to express myself and ask for what I need and want.
BLUE CHEESE SALAD DRESSING (on crispy greens)	Frustrated; feeling that there is no escape. Much blame toward self and others. Depression.	I have decided to take charge of following my inner dreams. I deserve the best.

BREAD (includes bagels, biscuits, muffins, rice cakes, pancakes, pastries, and waffles):

Toasted (crunchy):

Plain	Feeling like progress is thwarted. Frustrated.	I move toward my goals with trust and steady effort.
With butter	Feeling trapped, and procrastinating about making necessary changes.	I am free to make changes and pursue my Divinely inspired dreams.
With banana	Frustrated and depressed. Wanting a miraculous breakthrough.	The true source of inspiration is inside of me. I am provided with all the answers I need.
With cheese	Anxious about reaching goals and depressed about the future.	I trust my inner voice and follow its wisdom and direction.

Food Craved	Probable Meaning	Affirmation
With chocolate	Desiring love, support, and encouragement.	I am strong, loved, and supported.
With cinnamon	Feeling alone or abandoned. Too much to do, and not enough help.	I am warmed, knowing that I am enveloped in love. I radiate love outward, and all my needs are abundantly taken care of.
With garlic (garlic bread)	Desiring escape from an overly intense situation.	I release all my fears and replace them with strength and renewal.
With honey	Unsure whether you are equipped to take on a task or make necessary changes.	I have the time, talent, and intelligence to accomplish all my desires.
With jam, jelly, or syrup	Tired and overwhelmed. Desiring relief and energy.	I am renewed in mind, body, and spirit. When I follow my inner voice, my enthusiasm is boundless.
With meat, fowl, fish, or lox	Tired and desiring a wave of renewed energy. Frustrated or discouraged.	I bathe my spirit with the refreshing energy of love and self-approval.
With peanut butter, smooth	Tired of not having enough fun. Fed-up with always putting self last.	I give myself permission to relax and let go, right now. I deserve to have fun.

Food Craved	Probable Meaning	Affirmation
BREAD, <u>Toasted</u>, cont'd.		
With peanut butter, crunchy	Angry at heavy workload, feeling that everyone but you is relaxing and having fun.	I have the right to ask for help and to take time out when I need it. I am self-loving when I take care of my need to relax and have fun.
With pesto	Frustrated at the lack of excitement and fun in one's life.	I am excited by the process of fulfilling my Divine purpose. I am filled with love.
<u>Untoasted (soft):</u>	Insecure and desiring comfort and reassurance.	I am safe and secure. Love is in me and surrounding me.
With banana	Feeling alone, afraid, and depressed.	I love myself and know I am never alone when my heart is filled with love. I allow myself to feel good.
With butter	Frightened of making necessary changes or taking action. Procrastinating and waiting until you feel more prepared.	I trust in the Divine creator who is sowing His plans through me. I know that He will support me completely as I carry out His will.
With cheese	Fear and Shame. Don't like present situation and afraid to move forward. Fear of failure.	I am always a success when I allow my inner voice to direct me. I trust that I am Divinely guided.
With chocolate	Wanting a love relationship to comfort you.	Love is reflected in me and around me. I now attract loving people into my life.

Food Craved	Probable Meaning	Affirmation
With cinnamon	Fear and shame. Feeling cold and alone; wanting comfort and love.	My inner warmth radiates and attracts. My Divine source of love never leaves me. I take action to fulfill my peace of mind.
With garlic (garlic bread)	Feeling bored and left out. Resentment from feeling excluded.	I am reassured by the knowledge that I am Divinely guided. I am right where I need to be.
With honey	Insecure. Fear of rejection, embarrassment, or abandonment.	I am safe, secure, and loved.
With jam, jelly, or syrup	Anger. Hurt feelings. Exhausted. Desire for comfort and energy.	I tap into my unlimited source of energy and self-love.
With meat, fowl, fish, or lox	Drained and desiring recharged batteries and emotional support.	I take excellent care of myself in all ways.
With peanut butter, smooth	I give myself permission to relax and play. Other people respond lovingly to my requests for help.	Depressed and upset that others are having fun without you. Self-pity.
With peanut butter, crunchy	A belief that there is a lack of time. Upset over being pushed hard, with no fun.	All my priorities are in order. I take a deep breath and gently restore my peace of mind. I look for, and see, humor in my situation.

Food Craved	Probable Meaning	Affirmation
BREAD, <u>Untoasted</u>, cont'd.		
With pesto	Feeling bored and fed up.	I create excitement in my life in healthy, loving ways.
BROWNIES (see "Chocolate")		
BURRITOS (see "Mexican food")		
BUTTERMILK	Desiring energy and reassurance. Distress at having to face a difficult situation.	I center myself in the place within filled with strength and harmony. I go to that place whenever I face a trying circumstance.
BUTTERMILK BISCUITS (see "Bread")		
BUTTERMILK PANCAKES (see "Bread")		
BUTTERMILK RANCH SALAD DRESSING	Tension. Wanting to relax and feel pleasant enjoyment. May feel sad or lonely.	I am surrounded by Divine sources of pleasure, comfort, and companionship.
CAKE		
Angel food or vanilla	Wanting to escape a frightening or stressful situation.	I know the true source of my power. I relax with the knowledge that my Divine intelligence can be trusted.
Apple-cinnamon	Feeling lonely, withdrawn. Regret, self-blame, and guilt. Wanting forgiveness and relief.	I feel good about being who I am. I know that I deserve love and understanding.

Food Craved	Probable Meaning	Affirmation
Carrot cake	Insecure and worried, either about your job or a family member.	I face necessary changes with trust, strength, and intelligence. I treat myself gently.
Chocolate	Feeling insecure, possibly due to relationship problems.	I trust that when I act in love, I am Divinely guided. I am humble and sincere in all my interactions with others.
Chocolate chip	Upset about problems in a relationship. Unsettled by a misunderstanding and harsh words.	I am soothed with the knowledge that I am never alone. I remain open to love, and am Divinely directed about my love life.
Chocolate fudge	Desiring escape and a harmonious union with a loved one. Strong desire for love and comfort.	I reap what I sow, and I am now sowing love in my life. I see the truth in everyone I meet, and know that we are all God's man-ifestations of love.
Chocolate with nuts	Wanting more free time, vacations, or nights on the town. Frustrated by lack of love and fun.	I have made a decision to enjoy my life. As I am learning to let go and trust God's plans, I am rewarded with joy and love.
Coconut	Anxious because of heavy workload with no end in sight.	I practice self-love when I set a realistic schedule for myself. I allow myself breaks and rest time.

Food Craved	Probable Meaning	Affirmation
CAKE, cont'd.		
Coffee cake	Fear. Feeling alone. Desire for warm friendship, love, and understanding.	I am enveloped in the warm embrace of reassuring love. My Divine source completely understands and takes care of my needs.
German chocolate	Anxious due to a belief that a lack of fun would be cured by the presence of a great love relationship.	I release my need to predict and control. I know that all is well in my life.
Pound or shortcake	Wanting to block out awareness of a painful reality. Fear of making a wrong decision.	I have the inner strength to carry on. I act with firm conviction and make my decisions based on love and wisdom.
Tira misu	Desire to shed the nerve-wracking tension and replace it with a refreshing wave of energy.	I bathe my soul with cleansing thoughts. My true source of energy begins with my peace of mind.
CANDY		
Almond Joy	Anger. Bored and angry or anxious about not having enough fun in love life.	I have the right to relax and have fun. I enjoy this moment now.
Butterfingers	A desire for friendship and fun, but afraid of rejection.	My friends are loving, fun people who accept me for who I am right now.

Food Craved	Probable Meaning	Affirmation
Caramel	Anxious and drained from excess nervous energy.	I give myself permission to take some time out and listen to my inner voice.
Chocolate chips	Angry that love life is unsatisfactory. Blaming self or others.	My inner source of love is expressing itself perfectly right this very minute; I listen and trust.

Chocolate-covered:

Cherries	A desire to relax in a comfortable love relationship.	All my fears are melting as I fall in love with my Divinely guided life.
Coconut	A desire for love and fun. Envy or jealousy.	My Divine source of pleasure is inside of me. I give and receive love with pleasure.
Liqueur	Wanting to block out fears about love life. Desiring comfort and companionship.	As I receive Divine guidance about my life, it is easy for me to release fears and control.
Peanut butter	A desire to have more fun in your love life. Wanting nights out, vacations, or dates.	I follow my heart toward fun and find that the childlike spirit is the true source of love.
Nuts	Frustrated because your love life is boring or nonexistent. Losing patience.	I have the right to plan my life and take charge of fulfilling my needs.

Food Craved	Probable Meaning	Affirmation
CANDY, Chocolate-covered, cont'd.		
Raisins	Upset that some part of your love life is unsettled or unacceptable.	I see clearly what needs to be done. I am open to honest discussion and clear communication.
Nestle's Crunch	Frustrated that your love partner does not agree with you.	I trust that my love is continuous and complete. I release the need to control and predict.
English toffee	Tension. A desire for complete comfort and frustration with respect to struggles.	I let go of the need to defend. I am safe and exist without apology.
Fudge, chocolate	An intense craving for love, and feeling an extreme desire for a good relationship.	I am centered and I radiate love. My peace of mind attracts loving people into my life.
Fudge with nuts	Wrestling with questions about your love life. You are unhappy, and resent the way you are treated. But you worry, "Is it okay for me to feel this way?"	All my experiences and feelings are valid. I have the right to express my feelings to myself and others. I deserve fun and love.
Good 'n' Plenty	You feel drained because something worries you. Fear of loss.	I take action where warranted, and channel worry into free-flowing meditation. Everything has a purpose.

Food Craved	Probable Meaning	Affirmation
Gumdrops	A gnawing worry that haunts you. You want to feel good about it.	I know, deep down, that my true beliefs will guide me. I am responsible for listening to this voice.
Hard candy, sweet	Resentment and a block against future prosperity. A desire for revenge.	I take time to listen to my true voice of reason. I release the need to have any problems, and I revel in the joy of prosperity.
Hard candy, hot	Frustrated that others aren't recognizing your talents and value. Not knowing how to gain recognition.	I create my own time line for creative recognition. I embrace my free time as an opportunity to learn and grow.
Jelly beans (in general)	Worries and insecurity about work, desperately seeking solutions.	Every one of my needs always has been, and always will be, taken care of.
Jelly beans, red-hot	Frustrated that you're not having enough excitement or recognition.	I deserve the attention and companionship of others.
Jelly beans, licorice	Frustration about lack of excitement is leading to draining feelings. Desiring energy.	Right now, I feel renewed and recharged. My source of true enthusiasm is within me.
Kit Kat	Your decision not to settle for the wrong mate or inappropriate behavior leaves you feeling lonely or abandoned.	I approach my love life with intelligence, grace, and love.

Food Craved	Probable Meaning	Affirmation
CANDY, cont'd.		
M&M's	Work is interfering with your desire to relax and get closer to your mate.	When I let go, all my relationships improve.
M&M's, peanut	Your love life feels boring, and you are angry.	I have fun and love in my life right this very moment.
Peppermint chocolate	Feeling drained because of a contentious relationship; wanting energy and love.	I am right; a great love relationship is energizing and refreshing me. I am now in love.
Peanut brittle	Feeling angry or resentful that life is dull or difficult. Feeling like others are blaming you.	I release all beliefs of fighting or difficulties, and affirm the truth of life's lightness and harmony.
Reese's peanut butter cups	Fear. Wanting more love and fun in your life. Desires for carefree romance.	Today, I become as a child and adopt an innocent anticipation of fun and freedom.
Snicker's	A desire for your love partner to understand your needs. Longing for carefree love, fun, and romance.	I open my heart and connect with my love partner. I drop all defenses and enjoy our togetherness.
Three Musketeers	Tension. Upset about a relationship, and confused about how to resolve the problem.	Divine wisdom speaks through me, and my mind stays centered on love.
Truffles, plain	Wanting to escape to a pure state of love and bliss.	I am love, and I am in love now.

Food Craved	Probable Meaning	Affirmation
Truffles with nuts	A deep longing for a storybook romance; wanting to be swept off one's feet.	Perfect love resides within me now. I am complete and I am loved.
CEREAL, sweetened	Dreading upcoming tasks. Desiring energy and change of circumstance.	I make positive changes when needed. My inner voice always directs me.
Cap'n Crunch, peanut butter	Resentment over duties or chores. A desire to escape and be free to have more fun.	I follow my inner voice's direction toward goals that I naturally enjoy. I balance my life with regularly scheduled free time.
Cocoa Puffs	Tension. A belief that something is missing, and a desire for more love in one's life.	I relax and allow love to flow through me.
CEREAL, unsweetened		
Granola	Going through the motion of one's duties with resistance or resentment. Discouraged or depressed.	My purpose is Divinely guided. I listen to, and follow, my inner voice. I embrace changes that bring me closer to God.
Cream of wheat (also see "Oatmeal")	A desire for reassurance and support. Wanting comfort for sadness.	I am open to receiving love from others. I notice small examples of human kindness.
CHEESE (also see the food that the cheese is served on — e.g., pizza, nachos, etc.)	Braced for the worst, and feeling exhausted and drained. A desire for comfort and renewal. Thoughts centered on fear or worst-case scenarios. Weariness.	My source of energy shines brightly within me. I replace thoughts of fear with feelings of love.

Food Craved	Probable Meaning	Affirmation
CHEESECAKE		
Chocolate	Fears concerning a love relationship. A desire to be loved and appreciated.	I am comforted by my inner source of love.
Plain	Fears are triggering some feelings of depression. Wanting reassurance.	I focus on trusting the Divine wisdom within me. I know that I am guided, and I listen.
With fruit	Wanting reassurance and a fresh start. A desire to wipe the slate clean.	Today, I begin a new day and spend each moment in purpose and love.
With nuts	A desire for friendship and fun. Wanting closeness with others.	I am a good friend to myself and others. My friends are loving people.
CHEESE LOG ROLLED WITH NUTS	Wanting stimulation. Reluctance or guilt about having fun.	I embrace today and welcome each opportunity to connect with others.
CHICKEN (and all poultry)		
Ala King	Tension. Wanting comfort and energy, feeling drained or depressed.	I am renewed and ready to fulfill my inner vision. I know the right thing to do.
Baked, broiled, or roasted	A desire for parental love, harmony in the family, and simplicity.	My Divine parent warms my heart and my life with guidance, love, and complete support.
Barbecued, crispy	Wanting relaxation and time out.	I have the right to relax and enjoy myself.

Food Craved	Probable Meaning	Affirmation
Buffalo wings (spicy)	A desire to let go of cares and have an exciting time.	Everything in my life is perfect right now. I give all my cares and worries to God.
Cacciatore or parmigiana	Some frustration is creating an energy drain or depression.	I let go of trying to force a solution. I know all the answers I seek are within me. When I relax and trust, all my questions are answered.
Crispy fried	Feeling goals are thwarted and tired of encountering many roadblocks.	I take a quiet moment to assess my goals. I ask myself, "What is my gut feeling about this situation?"
With dumplings	Wanting validation, solace, and reassurance.	When I follow my gut feelings and act in accordance, I am rewarded with peace of mind.
Fried (moist)	Self-blame and fear of repercussions. Feeling alone and defenseless.	I am filled with faith and love. I ask for guidance in correcting my thinking about this situation. I forgive myself and let it go.
Pot pie	Wanting to block out thoughts of problems. Desiring escape and comfort.	I give myself permission to put my worries on the shelf for the evening. I will know what to do.
With rice (American style)	Tension. Desire to feel lighthearted and carefree.	A breath of spring blows through me, whisking away my cares. I am refreshed and renewed.

Food Craved	Probable Meaning	Affirmation
CHICKEN, cont'd.		
With rice (Mexican style)	Desire for relief from pressure. Life feels complicated and devoid of pleasure.	I release the need to plan and control the outcome. I stay focused on serving God.
CHICKEN SOUP WITH NOODLES AND RICE	Wanting to be soothed and comforted. Feeling hurt or misunderstood.	I focus on the gentle glow of love in my heart and ask it to radiate through me with healing warmth. My burdens are lifted.
CHILI	Wanting excitement and an outlet for stress.	I release my old ideas about how my life is supposed to look. My life is now changing in exciting ways, and I embrace this source of joy.
CHILI WITH CHEESE AND/OR SOUR CREAM	Anger and tension. Stress has built up to the point where you can't see any light at the end of the tunnel. This makes you feel down or depressed, and you long for fun, excitement, and change.	What a relief it is to relax and let go! As I clear away the fog of fear, I am given a clear vision of what I need to do. My life is filled with meaning and joy.
CHIPS (potato or corn)	You feel stressed or anxious, and you want to ease your worry. Also, a desire for validation.	I am willing to trust that everything works out for the best. I let go of feeling responsible for everything and everyone around me.
Spicy	Overwhelmed with too many dull and boring responsibilities.	I am open to receiving the lesson in this situation. I follow my joy.

Food Craved	Probable Meaning	Affirmation
With dip or cheese	Anger and tension. Anxiety or anger that has turned into depression. Self-anger or feeling betrayed.	I now realize I am Divinely directed. When I focus on love and joy, I am automatically led away from any source of pain or hurt.
With salsa	Tension. You are in a monotonous situation and long for more meaningful or exciting work. Frustration.	I deserve to realize my dreams, which will ultimately make the world a better place. I am ready for changes now.

CHOCOLATE
(see appropriate food category: candy, ice cream, cake, doughnut)

COFFEE	Energy drain from engaging in activities that are meaningless or intimidating to you. Burnout, resentment, or disappointment with your job.	I center my thoughts on the true source of energy, truth, and guidance deep inside me.
COLA, DIET	A desire to feel full and energized. Also, a wish for exciting romantic feelings.	Love fills me through and through.
COLA, REGULAR	You are trying to stay motivated and energized, and you are combatting internal stress.	When I follow my inner voice, all my needs are supplied.

CONDIMENTS

Butter	Procrastination. Resistance to fulfilling one's inner dreams.	I listen to, trust, and follow God's direction.
Catsup	Desire to be carefree as a child and feel high-energy playfulness.	I embrace pleasure and spread my joy.

Food Craved	Probable Meaning	Affirmation
CONDIMENTS, cont'd.		
Mayonnaise	Trepidation or insecurity about what you are doing. Desire for support and guidance.	I listen to, and let go of, my resistance and know that I am Divinely supported.
Mustard	Desire to rise above a mundane or disappointing situation. Judging or resenting others.	I change my outer world when I change my desires and beliefs.
COOKIES		
Almond, Chinese	Wanting to escape through a fun, yet comfortable activity.	I give myself permission to enjoy myself in all my activities.
Animal	Tension. A desire for more play time. Feeling a need for rewards and appreciation.	I delight in my innocence and encourage the child within me to express joy through play.
Batter, uncooked	Feeling vulnerable to attack from others. Also, angry at self.	It is safe to express my true feelings; I forgive and I love.
Butter cookies	Procrastination. A desire for peace of mind and comfort.	All my cares are melting away, and my heart is now filled with love.
Chocolate	Tension and fear. Braced for relationship problems. Aching for love.	I release this problem to you, dear Lord. You know what I need better than I do.
Chocolate chip, crunchy	Tension and anger. Irritated at love partner.	I open my heart to forgiveness so I can heal this relationship.
Chocolate chip, soft	Frightened that love relationship may be irreparably damaged. Fear of change or rejection.	I let go and trust that my life is changing for the better.

Food Craved	Probable Meaning	Affirmation
Chocolate chip, with nuts	Tension and fear. Upset that love relationship is unfulfilling.	I now seek avenues to increase the love in my life. I attract wonderful, loving people.
Cinnamon	Feeling cold and lonely. Frightened of the future.	When I surrender my life to God, only good can happen.
Fortune	Braced for problems.	I expect only the best, and that's what I receive.
Gingerbread	A desire for simplicity.	My life is clear and full of joy.
Lemon	Tension. A desire for friendship.	My friends are loving people who reflect my values and beliefs.
Oatmeal	Wanting direction in making a decision.	The source of my answers is within me. All I have to do is ask and then listen.
Oreos	Tension and shame. Punishing self for perceived lack of love.	I have decided to put my life back on course, and am rewarded with abundance and love.
Peanut butter, crunchy	Tension. Frustrated by a lack of fun.	I am redesigning my life, and it is beautiful and filled with joy.
Peanut butter, soft	Feeling guilty for relaxing, yet feeling sad because life isn't fun.	Fun is my Divine right. I now fulfill my need for joy and renewal.
Shortbread (see "Butter cookies")		
Sugar	Tension and fear. Wanting to hide from stress and problems. Procrastinating instead of taking action.	I am safe and secure.

Food Craved	Probable Meaning	Affirmation
CRACKER JACKS	Resentment because others are interfering with your pleasure.	All my actions reflect my higher self, and I express my needs with love.
CRACKERS (see "Salty Snacks")		
DOUGHNUTS		
Apple-cinnamon	A desire for motivation. Dread and trepidation.	I know the truth about this situation and am willing to make needed changes.
Chocolate	Anger. Disappointment over love life. Feeling betrayed, and desiring comfort.	My soul is soothed as I prepare to accept love into my life.
Glazed	Drained from being constantly on guard.	I release my life into the loving arms of my Divine Creator. I ask for, and receive, His protection.
Jelly doughnuts	Drained by chronic stress and wanting renewed joy and energy.	I take refuge in my daily silent meditations where I realign my thoughts with what is true.
With nuts	Desire to replace stress with a carefree life. Resentment or bitterness.	I release blame and accept good graciously. I give and receive joy.
FISH/SHELLFISH		
Baked/broiled	Energy drain from stress.	I take time out to reflect and recharge myself.
Deep-fried	Feeling pushed or overworked.	I have decided to make some changes, and that decision provides relief and solutions.

Food Craved	Probable Meaning	Affirmation
Raw	Wanting escape and a new perspective.	I look at my life from all angles, and my creativity is released.
Tuna fish salad	Stressed or worried, and wanting to feel secure.	I stay focused on my inner vision, and in this way I am able to withstand storms.

FISH/SHELLFISH, with:

Food Craved	Probable Meaning	Affirmation
Butter, melted	Wanting to feel sure of yourself before beginning an important project. Procrastination stemming from insecurity.	I am filled with the strength of love's direction.
Chips, soft/rice/ potatoes/pasta	Energy drain from excessive worrying. Wanting to feel grounded and secure.	I am comforted when I release my cares to God. He knows the perfect answer to my cares.
Crunchy chips	Nervousness and concern about outcome.	I take a deep breath and say a prayer, knowing that my peace of mind creates positive outcomes.
Spicy/Cajun/Thai	Pressure-cooker or high-risk job drains your energy. Desire to relax and feel certain.	My enthusiasm is high, and I enjoy learning from my challenges.
With white sauce	Feeling down or discouraged. Strong desires for comfort and energy; fear of staying discouraged. (This fear perpetuates the discouragement.)	I deserve the best in all areas of my life. I know that if I can dream it, I can do it.

Food Craved	Probable Meaning	Affirmation
FRENCH FRIES (see "Salty Snacks")		
FRITTER, DEEP FRIED	A desire for a simpler life; wanting to feel secure and return to one's roots.	I take my time and trust that solutions will present themselves to me. I slow down and stay open to observations of love.
FRUITS, crunchy	Tension. Stress-filled lifestyle is depleting your body's vitamins and minerals.	I nourish my body with love, and schedule time to meet my body's needs.
FRUITS, soft	Fear. Overattention to everyone else's needs, and not enough attention toward your own has depleted your body's vitamins and minerals.	I am important and deserve love. When I am healthy and happy, everyone benefits.
GRANOLA (see "Cereal")		
ICE CREAM (also see "Sherbet")		
Chocolate	Fear. Disappointment over love life, turned into depression or self-blame.	Deep down, I have an image of my true love life. I am following my inner guide's direction toward that love.
Chocolate chip	Fear and anger. Feeling angry that love life is unsatisfying, which triggers self-blame and depression.	I am comforted by knowing that I deserve love. I am open to receiving Divine guidance in all areas of my life.

Food Craved	Probable Meaning	Affirmation
Coffee	Feeling drained and wanting the desire to keep going.	I take a moment to examine my life, and I listen for direction about any needed changes. It is safe to start over.
Double chocolate chip	A feeling that love is being withheld or removed. Frustration that love partner won't change.	I now let go of fighting, and start anew with a soft heart. I bathe my soul in the cleansing comfort of kind thoughts.
English toffee/pralines	Upset that has turned into depression or a feeling of being wounded.	I look for a bright spot of humor in this situation, and am surprised how warmed I am by my own laughter.
French vanilla	Desire to feel secure and full.	I am filled with the comfort of God's love.
Fudgesicle	Feeling wounded by love life, and wanting a hug.	I ask for my needs to be met with love in my heart, and my request is always fulfilled when I am ready.
Mint chocolate chip	Feeling tired and frustrated because of many responsibilities and a perceived lack of love, time, money, or motivation.	I am renewed by the refreshing love I feel within me right now. I have enough time, energy, money, and motivation to accomplish all my desires.

Food Craved	Probable Meaning	Affirmation
ICE CREAM, cont'd.		
Peanut butter	Self-pity and disappointment. Lonely for friendship and fun.	I am a good friend and deserve the love of others. My friends and I have happy times together.
Pistachio	Wanting more fun in your life. Depressed that your responsibilities seem endless.	I clear a space in my heart for joy. My fun and joy begins inside me now.
Rocky road	Resentment toward others and self. Feeling used or pressured, and desiring fun and comfort. Depression.	I give and receive forgiveness, and my heart softens with love. This love then ensures that all my needs are met.
Strawberry	Wanting a fresh start with renewed enthusiasm.	Right now, my life is opening up to exciting new changes.
Vanilla	Tension and fear. Wanting to be soothed and renewed. Also, a desire for optimism.	I can decide right this minute to embrace the positive forces I feel inside of me.
ITALIAN FOOD		
Breadsticks (see "Bread")		
Calamari	Tension and fear. Anxious or worried and afraid to face the source of these feelings.	I face life head-on, feeling secure in the knowledge that my inner voice will guide me and keep me safe.
Calzone (see "Pizza")		

Food Craved	**Probable Meaning**	**Affirmation**
Cannelloni/ Manicotti/ Ravioli	Anger and shame. Feeling powerless to make needed changes. Feeling trapped and depressed in high-stress job.	I now reclaim my power and strength, which is fueled by truth and love.
Garlic bread (see "Bread")		
Lasagna	Trying to block awareness of emotional pain. A desire to shield oneself from attack.	My vulnerability is my greatest strength, because humility keeps me receptive to God's voice.
Pasta		
Plain	Wanting comfort and reassurance.	I fill my entire being with loving thoughts.
With Alfredo or extra cheese	Discouraged and wounded. Desire for empathy. Guilt or self-blame is blocking the receipt of good.	I graciously accept good into my life, knowing that I deserve pleasure, support and love.
With marinara	Resentment is causing distress.	I let go of all blame and focus on solutions.
With meat or fish	Wanting comfort and renewed energy.	My true source of energy comes from following my heart and inner guide.
With pesto	Wanting escape and excitement. Dreaming of time off or a vacation.	I decide to give myself a break and schedule some free time into my day.
With pine nuts	Feeling time pressures and resentment toward other. Wanting more fun.	Today, I look for moments of pleasure, fun, and enjoyment. I give myself the gift of laughter.

Food Craved	Probable Meaning	Affirmation
ITALIAN FOOD		
Pizza		
Crispy crust with:		
Extra cheese	Feeling afraid of the future. Reluctant or insecure.	I give myself permission to trust.
Extra meat	Feeling desperate for renewed energy or enthusiasm.	I am filled with enthusiasm for the fulfillment of my inner vision.
Spicy toppings/ anchovies	Tension, fear, and shame. Insecurity masked by workaholism. Drained from constant adrenaline highs.	I deserve the best in life. I face my dreams head-on, knowing that I deserve them.
"The works"	Drained from financial insecurities. Desire for abundance.	I now experience abundance in all areas of my life. God is a loving parent who wants the best for all His children.
Soft or regular crust with:		
Extra cheese	Depressed or discouraged, and wanting reassurance.	I am calmed by the presence of love deep inside of me. I feel warmed all over.
Extra meat	Energy drain from fears or insecurity.	I am good, I am safe, I am loved.
Spicy toppings/ anchovies	Confused and feeling out of touch with true feelings. Wanting pleasure and relief.	It is safe for me to enjoy myself.
"The works"	Struggling with lack in one's life. Feeling ripped off and yet having difficulty believing you deserve better.	I release the need to have lack in my life.

Food Craved	Probable Meaning	Affirmation

MEXICAN FOOD
   Crunchy Mexican Food (tacos, nachos, tostadas, etc.) with:

Food Craved	Probable Meaning	Affirmation
Extra cheese or sour cream	High stress in a mismatched job. Depression.	I have the right to make changes in my life. When I follow my inner guide, I am always safe.
Extra meat	Energy drain from futile struggles or an unworkable situation.	It is such a relief to let go of struggling! When I relax and trust, I am rewarded with peace of mind and abundance.
Extra salsa	Resentment and feeling trapped. Self-anger.	I have the right to change my life to fulfill my inner dreams.

   Soft Mexican Food (burritos, chili rellenos, etc.) with:

Food Craved	Probable Meaning	Affirmation
Extra cheese or sour cream	Feeling like a punching bag for others.	I have decided to surround myself with love. I am kind to myself, and others respond with respect toward me.
Extra meat	Despondent over feeling victimized.	I am victorious in fulfilling my Divine destiny. My present and future are bright and strong.
Extra salsa	Self-blame over unhappiness.	I ask for, and receive, respect and assistance.
NUTS	Tension. Too much stress and not enough fun—anxiety and lowered peace of mind.	It's okay for me to relax and play. I give myself permission to have fun.

Food Craved	Probable Meaning	Affirmation
ORIENTAL FOOD		
Almond chicken	Upset that life is all work and worries, and no fun or play.	I have the right to have fun, and to play. I give myself permission to schedule recreation into my life.
Crispy noodles	Stress and worry that a situation may backfire or result in a loss.	I am always safe and provided for.
Egg rolls	Desire to escape from all worries and stress.	I am comforted by my internal sanctuary, that place inside me filled with omnipotent wisdom and peace.
Kung pao dishes	Wanting more out of life, yet unsure of answers. Frustrated by too much work, and not enough rewards.	I take the time now to silently meditate. I ask my inner guide for answers, and I listen with an open heart.
Soft noodles	Wanting comfort and reassurance.	I fill my entire being with loving thoughts.
Soft noodles, spicy	Wanting more control. Trying to relax after a high-stress day.	I take deep breaths; I breathe out any cares or fears, and breathe in delicious feelings of renewal and relaxation.
Sushi/nori-maki	Tired of monotony; bored.	I follow my joy, and create a new life for myself.
Sweet and sour dishes	Fatigue from trying to do too many different things at once. Confusion. Desire for energy.	My life reflects order and peace.

Food Craved	**Probable Meaning**	**Affirmation**

PASTA (see "Italian Food")

PASTRY (see "Bread")

PEANUTS (see "Nuts")

PICKLES/ PICKLED FOODS	A desire for energy; stressed and drained.	I take time to renew myself with deep breaths, meditation, and time spent outdoors.

PIE

Apple	Self-blame or insecurity creates a desire to escape. Punishing oneself for perceived "wrongs."	I give myself a big hug. I Forgive, Accept, and Trust my Self.
Chocolate	Upset about love life: you don't have what you want, and are afraid you won't get the love you seek.	I have a clear and steady vision of what I want. I know that I deserve the best in all areas of my life.
Coconut	Anger. Wondering when you will have a good life. Envy or jealousy.	I am inspired by the success I see around me.
Fruit or berry	Wanting to start over. Regret is draining your energy.	I view every situation as an opportunity to learn and grow.
Peanut Butter	Desire for good, clean fun. Wanting old-fashioned friendships and activities.	Others like me, and I like them, too. I easily make friends with fun-loving people.

Food Craved	Probable Meaning	Affirmation
PIE, cont'd.		
Pecan	Feeling ripped off: Too much work and not enough rewards or fun.	I create a fun and fulfilling life for myself.
Pumpkin	Feeling afraid, lonely, or guilty and wanting to return to a time when you felt completely accepted.	I am safe, secure, and loved.
PIZZA (see "Italian Food")		
POPCORN		
With butter	Procrastinating starting a project, because of fears of failure.	If it's going to be, it's up to me. I trust and I push myself when necessary.
With caramel and nuts (Cracker Jacks)	Resentment because others are interfering with your pleasure.	All my actions reflect my higher self, and I express my needs with love.
PORK		
Bacon	Worries are draining your energy.	I trust that all the solutions I need are coming to me now.
Bacon, extra crispy	Too much stress in your life. Desire for energy and stamina to overcome troubling situation.	I am safe, and I now trust that all my needs are taken care of. I turn my worries over to God.
Chops, fried	Insecurity. Worry that situations will worsen.	My life is getting better with each moment. I am open to solutions.
Ribs	A high-stress day has left you desiring pleasure and calm.	The storm is over now, and my forecast calls for sunshine and peace in my life.

Food Craved	Probable Meaning	Affirmation
Sausage	Desire for energy and endurance to get through a difficult situation.	I call upon my inner source of strength, knowing that I have energy to see me through. I give myself permission to rest when needed.
Sausage, extra spicy	Desire for escape, wanting a vacation or exciting activity. Desire for attention and validation.	I listen to my needs and respond with love and kindness.

POTATO CHIPS (see "Chips")

POULTRY (see "Chicken")

PRETZELS	Tense. Strong desire to relax and let go of frustration.	I breathe deeply and let go for the moment.

PUDDING

Chocolate	A desire for comfort, nurturing, and hugs. Feeling vulnerable to the loss of love.	I have love here inside me. I give and receive love in my life.
Vanilla	Wanting a fresh start or a new perspective on a problem.	I see this situation in a new light of love.

SALTY SNACKS (also see "Chips" and "Bread")

Crackers	Tension. Indecision or trying to feel good about a situation that was thrust upon you.	This is important. I allow myself to breathe deeply and consider my situation.

Food Craved	Probable Meaning	Affirmation
SALTY SNACKS, Crackers, cont'd.		
With cheese or dip	Feeling depressed because an unwanted situation was forced or manipulated onto you.	I have the right to look at this situation and make my own decisions.
With peanut butter	Upset because you must work so much, when you'd rather be playing and having fun.	I enjoy this moment right now, and know that I am free.
With salsa	Upset because life seems routine and monotonous. You are craving some big-time excitement!	I find moments that excite me today; I enjoy the wonderful beauty of day-to-day life.
French fries, crisp	Tension, mixed with a sense of emptiness. Feeling as if you're missing the boat, and that there's something more meaningful you are meant to do.	I follow my gut feelings, which guide me in harmonious and meaningful directions.
French fries, soft	Depression and anxiety. You feel sad that your life doesn't match your dreams. A sense that you don't even want to attempt to fulfill your goals.	I am filled with the warm flow of love through my heart. I use this force to propel me toward my dreams, starting now.
Onion rings, crisp	Feeling stress from a change in your life, which makes you feel insecure.	I know that I am ready for the new challenges in my life. They make me grow stronger.
Onion rings, soft	Feeling sad that you've tried so hard, yet your companions or family don't seem to appreciate you. Loneliness.	I have a private relationship with God. He gives me Divine guidance, and I follow His direction.

Food Craved	Probable Meaning	Affirmation
SHERBET	A desire to unwind or celebrate.	I shed all worries, and replace them with jubilation.
TEA	Good intentions mixed with mistrust; creating blocks to intimacy and an energy drain.	All barriers to good are removed when I let go and trust.
TOAST (see "Bread")		
TOSTADA (see "Mexican food")		
TRUFFLES (see "Candy")		
VANILLA (see appropriate category— e.g., candy, ice cream, etc.)		
VEGETABLES, crispy	Tension. Stress-filled lifestyle is depleting body's vitamins and minerals.	I nourish my body with love, and schedule time to meet my body's needs.
VEGETABLES, soft	Fear. Overattention to everyone else's needs, and not enough attention toward your own has depleted your body's vitamins and minerals.	I am important and deserve love. When I am healthy and happy, everyone benefits.
WALNUTS (see "Nuts")		
YOGURT (for frozen yogurt, see "Ice Cream")	Feeling stuck and wanting a push in the right direction. Some depression because of self-compromise.	I give myself permission to correct and change my life.

Dear Reader,

I appreciate hearing about your experiences. Would you please take a moment to tell me a little about yourself. On a separate piece of paper:

1. Please tell me your age and a little about your personal and professional background.

2. Have you ever listened to your gut feelings and had a positive experience? If yes, please describe.

3. Have you ignored your gut feelings and regretted it? If yes, please explain.

4. Please include any other comments, including any questions you have (all letters will be personally answered).

Thank You!

Doreen Virtue
c/o Hay House, Inc.
P.O. Box 5100
Carlsbad, CA 92018-5100

(**Note**: *References to supplements in this glossary do not imply a recommendation or an endorsement. If you are interested in supplementing your diet with amino acids, vitamins, or minerals, please consult your physician.*)

Acetocholine—A brain chemical, or neurotransmitter, important in the regulation of appetite, memory, and the sex drive. The precursors for acetocholine are choline and lecithin, which naturally appear in eggs, soy products, beef, milk, and cashews.

Amino Acids—The basic components of protein. When you eat protein, it breaks down into amino acids in your body. Amino acids are precursors, or catalysts, for other chemicals in the body. In particular, amino acids are important in the production of brain chemicals called *neurotransmitters*. These brain chemicals regulate our mood, energy levels, appetite, memory, and sex drive. "Essential" amino acids are manufactured as a result of the foods or supplements that we eat. "Nonessential" amino acids aren't as contingent upon our diets, since the body naturally produces them. Both types of amino acids—nonessential and essential—are equally important (the word *nonessential* unwittingly suggests that it's not as important as *essential*, but that's not the case).

Arginine—An amino acid often classified as "nonessential." However, the body is only able to manufacture a small amount of arginine on its own. For that reason, many scientists argue that arginine is an "essential" amino acid. Arginine is important in glucose metabolism, insulin production, and regulating blood cholesterol levels. It occurs naturally in nuts and chocolate.

Aspartic Acid—A nonessential amino acid important in regulating metabolism and energy levels. It is thought to increase stamina and reduce fatigue. As a nonessential amino acid, the body produces this substance on its own. A version of aspartic acid called *asparagine* is a component of protein. Aspartic acid combines with the amino acid, *citrulline,* to form arginine. Aspartame (NutraSweet) is composed of aspartic acid and phenylalanine.

Carnitine—A nonessential amino acid important in metabolizing any fat that you may eat. It also plays a role in reducing triglycerides. Women appear to have naturally lower levels of carnitine than men. As a nonessential amino acid, carnitine is naturally produced by the body. Vitamin C deficiencies can result in carnitine deficiencies.

Choline—A precursor for the neurotransmitter, acetocholine, which plays an important role in regulating the appetite, memory, and sex drive. Choline is found naturally in eggs, milk, beef, cashews, and soy products.

Cystine—A derivative of the amino acid, methionine. Cystine is important in the body's natural detoxification processes. It is also essential in metabolizing vitamin B-6, which is important in serotonin production. Cystine naturally occurs in beans, eggs, onions, and garlic.

Diphenylamine—A substance occurring naturally in chocolate. Diphenylamine appears to mimic the role of serotonin, leading to feelings of calm and serenity.

Dopamine—An excitatory (stimulating) neurotransmitter. Dopamine's precursor is tyrosine, which naturally occurs in aged cheese, bananas, beer, chocolate, pickled foods, sausage, vanilla, wine, and yogurt.

Epinephrine—An excitatory (stimulating) neurotransmitter, important in the regulation of energy. The amino acid precursors to epinephrine include tyramine and tyrosine, which occur naturally in aged cheese, bananas, beer, chocolate, pickled foods, sausage, vanilla, wine, and yogurt.

Glutamine—A nonessential amino acid that plays a role in protecting the body from alcohol's poisoning effects. Glutamine has also been linked to alleviating depression, improving mental functioning, and reducing the craving for alcohol. As a nonessential amino acid, the body naturally produces glutamine supplies; however, it is also available in supplements.

Glycine—A nonessential amino acid important in the body's healing processes, especially for skin and connective tissue. As a nonessential amino acid, the body naturally produces its own supply; however, it is also available in supplements.

Histamine—A byproduct of the amino acid, histidine, this vasodilator increases the pulse rate and decreases blood pressure. It is derived from the amino acid, histidine, which is found in aged cheese, pickled foods, liver, yeast, wine, and beer.

Histidine—An essential stimulating amino acid that produces histamine. Histidine occurs naturally in aged cheese, pickled foods, liver, yeast, wine, and beer.

Homeostasis—The body's regulatory system, which ensures that all vital processes are properly balanced. The body is driven to maintain a proper balance of the vital needs for food, liquid, shelter, temperature, and peace of mind.

Isoleucine—An essential amino acid found naturally in beef, chicken, fish, nuts, seeds, and soy products. The role that isoleucine plays in the body is not entirely clear; however, one study did identify an isoleucine deficiency in mentally and physically ill patients. This is a correlative study, and does not necessary mean a cause-and-effect situation.

Leucine—An essential amino acid found naturally in corn, eggs, nuts, cottage cheese, whole wheat, and brown rice. Interestingly enough, there is ample evidence that excessive leucine interferes with the metabolism of vitamin B-3. Leucine is related to phenylalanine, and may therefore share some stimulating properties.

Lysine—An essential amino acid often prescribed in the treatment of herpes simplex virus. Lysine influences the appetite in an unexpected way: if you are deficient in this amino acid, your appetite decreases and weight loss may occur. For that reason, pediatricians often recommend giving children lysine as an instrument in ensuring appetite and growth. Lysine occurs naturally in fish, chicken, beef, lamb, milk, cheese, and beans. Lysine competes with the amino acid, arginine (and usually loses), so foods such as these, which are high in both arginine and lysine, will not ensure that the body receives sufficient lysine: chocolate, carob, coconut, and peanuts.

MDMA—The name of a once-legal drug derived from phenylethylamine or PEA (the same chemical found in smaller quantities in chocolate). This drug was prescribed for embittered couples, because the drug replaces hostility with euphoria. Today, this drug is an illegal substance known as "Ecstasy."

Methionine—An essential amino acid important in the body's natural detoxification processes. It is an antioxidant when sufficient amounts of vitamin B-6 are in the body, and is found in beans, beef, chicken, fish, pork, seeds, eggs, onions, cottage cheese, and garlic.

Methylxanthine—The family of stimulants found naturally in cocoa, tea, coffee, and cola nuts. Caffeine, theophylline, and theobromine are the three forms of methylxanthine found in dietary forms.

Monoamine Oxidase (MAO)—Prescribed in therapies to inhibit the release of neurotransmitters, to relieve depression or anxiety. People prescribed with MAO are advised to avoid foods high in tyramine to avoid hypertension.

Neurotransmitter—The brain's chemical messengers, which are created by a brain cell's activity, and which, in turn, spark another brain cell's electrical currents, and brain activity. Neurotransmitters are either excitatory (stimulating) or inhibitory (calming).

Noradrenaline—An excitatory (stimulating) neurotransmitter important in energy regulation, and also influential in feelings of anxiety or panic. Tyramine is a precursor for noradrenaline, and tyramine occurs naturally in aged cheese, sausage, pickled foods, beer, and wine.

Norepinephrine—An excitatory (stimulating) neurotransmitter essential for energy, learning, and memory. Norepinephrine also helps brain cells to communicate with one another. This chemical is created from the amino acid, phenylalanine, and the precursors, tyramine and tyrosine. One study found that obese individuals have lower-than-normal levels of norepinephrine, as well as low serotonin. The precursors for norepinephrine occur naturally in aged cheese, bananas, beer, chocolate, pickled foods, sausage, vanilla, wine, and yogurt.

Phenylalanine—An essential stimulating amino acid found in high-protein foods such as dairy products, meat, and nuts. Phenylalanine converts into the stimulant tyrosine, which in turn triggers the production of the brain chemicals, dopamine, epinephrine, and norepinephrine. Phenylalanine accounts for one-half of the ingredients in aspartame ("NutraSweet"). The other half of NutraSweet is another stimulating amino acid called *aspartic acid*. There is some evidence that phenylalanine may trigger the production of the "Love Drug," phenylethylamine (PEA). Phenylalanine is also considered an appetite suppressant, since it triggers production of cholycystokinin (CCK).

CCK not only satisfies hunger, but also increases alertness and memory, alleviates depression, and increases the sex drive. Phenylalanine naturally occurs in soy products, nut, poultry, fish, meat, and cottage cheese.

Phenylethylamine (PEA)—The so-called Love Drug, which the brain produces during romantic situations. Two ounces of chocolate contains approximately 3 mg of PEA, in exactly the same form as the brain chemical. This chemical is a strong stimulant of the metha-amphetamine family. PEA was once prescribed as a drug known as MDMA, for couples who were contemplating divorce. The drug replaces hostility with temporary feelings of euphoria. Today, MDMA is an illegal street drug known as "Ecstasy."

Precursor—A catalyst in the creation of a neurotransmitter.

Psychoactive—Mood-altering; something that affects depression and anxiety levels. Psychoactive substances include food, alcohol, and medications such as antidepressants.

Pyrozine—A psychoactive chemical that triggers the brain's pleasure center and creates a pleasant, happy feeling. Pyrozine enters the brain through the olfactory system—in other words, through our nose. The smell of burnt nuts indicates the presence of pyrozine. It is found naturally in coffee, chocolate, nuts, and some colas.

Serotonin—An inhibitory (calming) neurotransmitter, important in the regulation of mood, energy levels, appetite, and sex drive. Serotonin is manufactured on a daily basis during the REM sleep cycle and cannot be stored. When serotonin is low, we feel depressed, irritable, lethargic, and hungry. Serotonin levels are affected by habits of sleep, eating, exercise, stress, alcohol, and drug consumption and personality.

Taurine—A nonessential calming amino acid, taurine is a precursor to the inhibitory (calming) neurotransmitters. Taurine helps the body maintain a balance of the other amino acids, and of the blood sugar levels. As a nonessential amino acid, taurine is produced in the body; however, it is also available in supplement form. Taurine production appears to hinge upon the body having a sufficient supply of the mineral, zinc.

Theobromine—A stimulant of the "xanthine" family, found naturally in tea, chocolate, and coffee. Chocolate contains an especially high percentage of theobromine.

Theothylline—The sister stimulant of theobromine, from the "xanthine" family. It, too, occurs naturally in tea, chocolate, and coffee.

Threonine—An essential calming amino acid important in mood regulation. Irritability and "difficult" personalities have been linked to threonine deficiencies. Threonine naturally occurs in cheese (especially cheddar and cottage cheese), fish, soy products, beef, lamb, pork, milk, and poultry.

Tryptophan—An essential calming amino acid derived from high-protein foods, including dairy products, meat, and poultry. Tryptophan is important in the production and maintenance of the brain neurotransmitter, serotonin. Therefore, tryptophan plays a role in depression and appetite, since low serotonin creates disorders in both realms. However, tryptophan does not compete well against other amino acids. Carbohydrates play an important role in diverting competing amino acids away from the blood brain barrier, so that tryptophan can enter the brain and trigger the production of serotonin. High quantities of tryptophan are found in dairy products, beef, poultry, pork, and fish.

Tyramine—A stimulant, derived from tyrosine, that raises blood pressure, found naturally in aged cheese, bananas, beer, chocolate, pickled foods, sausage, vanilla, wine, and yogurt. One of the most powerful vasoactive stimulants found naturally in food. Those on MAO antidepressant therapies, and highly sensitive individuals, can suffer from migraine headaches or hypertensive crises when they eat foods high in tyramine.

Tyrosine—A stimulant that produces tyramine, found naturally in aged cheese, chocolate, sausage, vanilla, beer, wine, and pickled foods. Tyrosine is a precursor, or agent, in the production of norepinephrine and epinephrine. Tyrosine is made from the amino acid, phenylalanine.

Valine—An essential amino acid naturally occurring in cottage cheese, fish, chicken, beef, lamb, nuts, brown rice, and soy products. Valine appears to play a role in appetite suppression, since it works with phenylalanine, methionine, and tryptophan in the production of the natural appetite suppressant known as *cholecystokinin* (CCK). However, researchers do not yet clearly understand valine's role in suppressing the appetite.

Vasoactive—Any substance that changes the blood pressure or pulse rate. Many amino acids found in foods and beverages are vasoactive in one of two ways: they are vasoconstrictors, which narrow the blood vessels and increase blood pressure; and vasodilators, which open the blood vessels and decrease blood pressure.

Xanthine—Another term for *methylxanthine,* which is the family of stimulants found naturally in cocoa, tea, coffee, and cola nuts. Caffeine, theophylline, and theobromine are the three forms of methylxanthine found in dietary forms.

CHAPTER ONE: Fat Is a Spiritual Issue

1. Lyman, B. (1989), *A Psychology of Food: More Than a Matter of Taste*. New York: AVI Publishing.

2. British Nutrition Foundation (1973), "Report on a Survey of Housewives' Knowledge and Attitudes." In: *Nutrition and Lifestyles*, Turner, M. (Ed.), pp. 157 - 158. London: Applied Science Publishers, Ltd.

   Jenkins, N. K. (1964), *Nutrition* (U.K.), Vol. 18, p. 115.

3. Dwyer, J. T., et al. (1967). *American Journal of Clinical Nutrition*, Vol. 20, p. 1045.

4. Thomas, J. (1979), "The Relationship Between Knowledge About Food and Nutrition and Food Choice." In: *Nutrition and Lifestyles*, Turner, M. (Ed.), pp. 141 - 167. London: Applied Science Pubs., Ltd.

CHAPTER TWO: The FATS Feelings

1. Plutchik, R. (1976), "Emotions and Attitudes Related to Being Overweight." *Journal of Clinical Psychology*, Vol. 32, pp. 21 - 24.

2. Goldsmith, S. J., et al. (1992), "Psychiatric Illness in Patients Presenting for Obesity Treatment." *International Journal of Eating Disorders*, Vol. 12 (1), pp. 63 - 71.

3. Slochower, J., et al. (1981), "The Effects of Life Stress and Weight on Mood and Eating." *Appetite*, Vol. 2, pp.115 - 125.

4. Strober, M. (1984), "Stressful Life Events Associated with Bulimia in Anorexia Nervosa." *International Journal of Eating Disorders*, Vol. 3, No. 2, pp. 3 - 15.

5. Slochower, J. and Kaplan, S.P. (1980), "Anxiety, Perceived Control, and Eating in Obese and Normal Weight Persons." *Appetite*, Vol. 1, pp. 75 - 83.

CHAPTER FIVE: Appetite: The Drive to Survive

1. Fomon, S. J., et al. (1971), "Food Consumption and Growth of Normal Infants Fed Milk-Based Formulas." *Acta Paediatrics* (Supp.), Vol. 223, p. 36.

Fomon, S. J., et al. (1969), "Relationship Between Formula Concentration and Rate of Growth of Normal Children." *Journal of Nutrition*, Vol. 98, pp. 241 - 254.

2. Ashworth, A. (1974), "Ad Lib. Feeding During Recovery from Malnutrition." *British Journal of Nutrition*, Vol. 31, pp. 109 - 112.

3. Foltin, R. W., et al. (1988), "Compensation for Caloric Dilution in Humans Given Unrestricted Access to Food in a Residential Laboratory," *Appetite*, Vol. 10, pp. 13 - 24.

4. Newsome, J. and Newsome, E. (1966) *Patterns of Infant Care*. New York: Penguin.

5. Birch, L. L. (1987), "Children's Food Preferences: Developmental Patterns and Environmental Influences." In: Vasta, R. (Ed.), *Annals of Child Development,* Vol. 4, Greenwich, CT: JAI Press.

Birch, L. L. and Deysher, M. (1985), "Conditioned and Unconditioned Caloric Compensation: Evidence for Self-Regulation of Food Intake in Young Children." *Learning and Motivation*, Vol. 16, pp. 341 - 355.

Birch, L. L., et al. (1982), "Effects of Instrumental Consumption on Children's Food Preference." *Appetite*, Vol. 3, pp. 125 - 134.

Birch, L. L. (1981), "Generalization of a Modified Food Preference." *Child Development*, Vol. 52, pp. 755- 758.

Birch, L. L., et al. (1980), "The Influence of Social-Affective Context on the Formation of Children's Food Preferences." *Child Development*, Vol. 51, pp. 856 - 861.

6. Cohen, I. T., et al. (1987), "Food Cravings, Mood and the Menstrual Cycle," *Hormones and Behavior*, Vol. 21, pp. 457 - 470.

Harvey, J., et al. (1993), "Effects on Food Cravings of a Very Low-Calorie Diet or a Balanced, Low-Calorie Diet." *Appetite*, Vol. 21, pp. 105 - 115.

Hill, A. J., et al. (1991), "Food Craving, Dietary Restraint and Mood." *Appetite*, Vol. 17, pp. 187 - 197.

Hill, A. J. and Blundell, J. E. (1990), "Sensitivity of the Appetite Control System in Obese Subjects to Nutritional and Serotoninergic Challenges." *International Journal of Obesity*, Vol. 14, pp. 219 - 233.

Rodin, J., et al. (1991), "Food Cravings in Relation to Body Mass Index, Restraint and Estradiol Levels: A Repeated Measures Study in Healthy Women." *Appetite*, Vol. 17, pp. 177 - 185.

Weingarten, H. P. and Elston, D. (1991), "Food Cravings in a College Population." *Appetite*, Vol. 17, pp. 167 - 175.

Weingarten, H. P. and Elston, D. (1990), "The Phenomenology of Food Cravings." *Appetite*, Vol. 15, pp. 231 - 246.

7. Berry, S. L., et al. (1985), "Sensory and Social Influences on Ice Cream Consumption by Males and Females in a Laboratory Setting." *Appetite*, Vol. 6, pp. 41 - 45.

   Edelman, B., et al. (1986), "Environmental Effects on the Intake of Overweight and Normal-Weight Men." *Appetite*, Vol. 7, pp. 71 - 83.

8. Galef, B. G., et al. (1987), "'Hungry Rats' Following of Conspecifics to Food Depends on the Diets Eaten by Potential Leaders." *Animal Behaviour* (U.K.) Vol. 35, pp. 1234 - 1239.

   Galef, B. G. and Wigmore, S. W. (1983), "Transfer of Information Concerning Distant Foods: A Laboratory Investigation of the 'Information Centre' Hypothesis." *Animal Behaviour* (U.K.), Vol. 13, pp. 748 - 758.

   Galef, B.G. (1977), "Mechanisms for the Social Transmission of Acquired Food Preferences from Adult to Weanling Rats." In: Barker, L. M., et al. (Eds.), *Learning Mechanisms in Food Selection*. Texas: Baylor University Press.

9. Kawai, M. (1965), "Newly Acquired Pre-Cultural Behavior of the Natural Troop of Japanese Monkeys on Koshima Islet." *Primates*, Vol. 6, pp. 1 - 30.

   Suboski, M. D. and Bartashunas, C. (1984), "Mechanisms for Social Transmission of Pecking Preferences to Neonatal Chicks." *Journal of Experimental Psychology*, Vol.10, pp. 182 - 194.

   Wyrwicka, W. (1981) *The Development of Food Preferences*. Springfield, IL: Charles C. Thomas Publishers.

10. Brobeck, J. R. (1948), "Food Intake as a Mechanism of Temperature Regulation." *Journal of Biology and Medicine*, Vol. 20, pp. 545 - 552.

11. Kraly, F. S. and Blass, E. M. (1976), "Increased Feeding in Rats in a Low Ambient Temperature." In: Novin, D., et al. (Eds.), *Hunger: Basic Mechanisms and Clinical Implications*. New York: Raven Press.

12. Galst, J. P. and White, M. A. (1976), "The Unhealthy Persuader: The Reinforcing Value of Television and Children's Purchase-Influencing Attempts at the Supermarket." *Child Development*, Vol. 47, pp. 1089-1096.

   Goldberg, M. E., et al. (1978), "TV Messages for Snack and Breakfast Foods: Do They Influence Children's Preferences?" *Journal of Consumer Research*, Vol. 5, pp. 73 - 81.

   Virtue, D. (1989), "Watch and Grow Thin," *T.V. Guide*, Vol. 37, No. 25, pp. 17 - 19.

13. Jeffrey, D. B., et al. (1982), "The Development of Children's Eating Habits: The Role of Television Commercials." *Health Education Quarterly*, Vol. 9, pp. 174 - 189.

Jeffrey, D. B., et al. (1980), "Television Food Commercials and Children's Eating Behavior: Some Emperical Evidence." *Journal of the University Film Association*, Vol. 32, pp. 41 - 43.

Jeffrey, D. B., et al. (1980), "The Impact of Television Advertising on Children's Eating Behaviour: An Integrative Review." *Catalog of Selected Documents in Psychology*, Vol. 10, No. 11, Ms. 2011.

14. Friedrich, J. A. (1987) *The Pre-Menstrual Solution*. San Jose: Arrow Press.

Wurtman, J. J. (1981), "Neurotransmitter Regulation of Protein and Carbohydrate Consumption." In: Miller, S.A. (Ed.), *Nutrition and Behavior*. Philadelphia: Franklin Institute.

Wurtman, R. J. (1988), "Effects of Their Nutrient Precursors on the Synthesis and Release of Serotonin, the Catecholamines, and Acetylcholine: Implications for Behavioral Disorders." *Clinical Neurophramacology*, Vol. 11 (Supp. 1), pp. S187 - S193.

15. Uvnas-Moberg (1989), "Gastrointestinal Tract in Growth and Reproduction." *Scientific American*, Vol. 261, pp. 78 - 83.

16. Hook, J. S. (1978), "Dietary Cravings and Aversions During Pregnancy." *The American Journal of Clinical Nutrition*, Vol. 31, pp. 1355 - 1362.

17. Buist, R. (1988), *Food Chemical Sensitivity*. Garden City Park, NY: Avery Publishing Group.

Lavin, M. J., et al. (1980), "Transferred Flavor Aversions in Adult Rats." *Behavioral and Neural Biology*, Vol. 28, pp. 15 - 33.

Revusky, S., et al. (1980), "Unconditioned Stimulus Preexposure: Effects on Flavor Aversions Produced by Pairing a Poisoned Partner with Ingestion." *Animal Learning and Behavior*, Vol. 10, pp. 83 - 90.

18. Clay, K. (1989), "Trespassers Will Be Poisoned." *Natural History* (Sept.), pp. 8 - 14.

Logue, A. W. (1979), "Taste Aversion and the Generality of the Laws of Learning." *Psychological Bulletin*, Vol. 86, pp. 276 - 296.

Rozin, P. and Kalat, J. W. (1971), "Specific Hungers and Poison Avoidance as Adaptive Specializations of Learning." *Psychological Review*, Vol. 78, pp. 459 - 486.

CHAPTER SIX: Why Do We Eat More at Buffets?

1. Davis, C. M. (1939), "Results of the Self-Selection of Diets by Young Children." *The Canadian Medical Association Journal*, pp. 257 - 261.

   Davis, C. M. (1930) *Can Babies Choose Their Food?* The Parents' Magazine, Vol. 22. pp. 42 - 43.

   Davis, C. M. (1928), "Self-Selection of Diets by Newly Weaned Infants." *American Journal of Disease of Children*, Vol. 36, pp. 651 - 679.

2. Halliday, A. W. and Halliday, J. W. (1994) *Silent Hunger*. Grand Rapids, MI: Revell/Baker Book House.

3. Richter, C. P., et al. (1938) *American Journal of Physiology*, Vol. 122, pp. 734 - 744.

4. LeMagnen, J. (1985) *Hunger*. Cambridge, Great Britain: Cambridge University Press.

   Rolls, B., Rowe, E. and Rolls, E. (1980), "Appetite and Obesity: Influences of Sensory Stimuli and External Cues." In: Turner, M. (Ed.), *Nutrition and Lifestyles*, pp. 11 - 19. Essex, England: Applied Science Publishers.

5. Rolls, B. J., et al. (1981), "Variety in a Meal Enhances Food Intake in Man."*Physiology and Behavior*, Vol. 26, pp. 215 - 221.

6. Rolls, B., Rowe, E. and Rolls, E. (1980), Op. cit.

7. Rolls, B., Rowe, E. and Rolls, E. (1980), Ibid.

8. Holling, C. S. (1965) *Mem. Ent. Society* (Canada), Vol. 45, p. 60.

   Kear, J. A. (1962) *Procedures of the Zoological Society*, London, Vol. 138, pp. 163 - 204.

   Morrison, G. R. (1974) *Journal of Comprehensive Physiological Psychology*, Vol. 86, pp. 56 - 61.

   Rolls, B., Rowe, E. and Rolls, E. (1980), Op. cit.

   Young, P. T. (1940) *Journal of General Psychology*, Vol. 22, pp. 33 - 66.

9. Rogers, Q. R. and Leung, P.M.B. (1977), "The Control of Food Intake: When and How Are Amino Acids Involved?" In: Kare, M.R. and Maller, O. (Eds.), *The Chemical Senses and Nutrition*. New York: Academic Press.

   Rozin, P. (1976), "The Selection of Foods by Rats, Humans and Other Animals." In: Rosenblatt, J.S., et al. (Eds.), *Advances in the Study of Behavior*, Vol. 6. New York: Academic Press.

Rozin, P. (1972), "Specific Aversions as a Component of Specific Hungers." In: Seligman, M.E.P. and Hager, J. L. (Eds.), *Biological Boundaries of Learning*. New York: Appelton-Century-Crofts.

Zahorik, D.M. and Houpt, K.A. (1977), "The Concept of Nutritional Wisdom: Applicability of Laboratory Learning Models to Large Herbivores." In: Barker, L.M., et al. (Eds.) *Learning Mechanisms in Food Selection*. Texas: Baylor University Press.

Zahorik, D.M. and Maier, S. F. (1972), "Appetitive Conditioning with Recovery from Thiamine Deficiency as the Unconditional Stimulus." In: Seligman, M.E.P. and Hager, J. L. (Eds.) *Biological Boundaries of Learning*. New York: Appleton-Century-Crofts.

CHAPTER SEVEN: How Your Personality Affects Your Weight

1. Rodin, J. (1980), "The Externality Theory Today." In: Stunkard, A. J. (Ed.) *Obesity*. Philadelphia: Saunders.

2. Watson, R. (1980), "Psychological Influences on Eating Behavior." In: Turner, M. (Ed.), *Nutrition and Lifestyles*, pp. 43 - 52. London: Applied Science Publishers, Ltd.

3. Watson, R. (1980), Op. cit.

4. Rodin, J. and Slochower, J. (1976) *Journal of Personality and Social Psychology*, Vol. 33, pp. 338 - 344.

5. Rodin, J., et al. (1985), "Effect of Insulin and Glucose on Feeding Behavior."*Metabolism*, Vol. 34, pp. 826 - 831.

6. Lyman, B. (1989), Op. cit.

CHAPTER EIGHT: How Foods Change Our Moods

1. Conners, C.K. and Blouin, A. G. (1983), "Nutritional Effects on Behavior of Children." *Journal of Psychiatric Research*, Vol. 17, pp. 193 - 201.

   Pollitt, et al. (1983), "Fasting and Cognitive Function." *Journal of Psychiatric Research*, Vol. 17, pp. 169 - 174.

2. Turkewitz, G. (1975), "Learning in Chronically Protein-Deprived Rats." In: Serban, G. (Ed.), *Nutrition and Mental Functions*, New York: Plenum Publishing.

   Zimmermann, R. R., et al. (1975), "Behavioral Deficiencies in Protein-Deprived Monkeys." In: Serban, G. (Ed.), *Nutrition and Mental Functions*, New York: Plenum Publishing.

3. Greenwood, C. and Winocur, G. (1994), "Toronto Researchers Say a High-Fat Diet May Dull the Brain." *Orange County Register*, December 16.

    Leibel, R. L., et al. (1981), "Methodological Problems in the Assessment of Nutrition-Behavior Interactions: A Study of Effects of Iron Deficiency on Cognitive Function in Children." In: Miller, S. A. (Ed.), *Nutrition and Behavior*. Philadelphia: Franklin Institute.

4. Buist, R. (1988), Op. cit.

    Pennington, J.A.T. and Church, H. N. (1985) *Food Values of Portions Commonly Used*. New York: Harper and Row.

5. King, D. S. (1981), "Food and Chemical Sensitivities Can Produce Cognitive-Emotional Symptoms." In: Miller, S. A. (Ed.), *Nutrition and Behavior*, Philadelphia: Franklin Institute.

6. Henriksen, S., et al. (1974), "The Role of Serotonin in the Regulation of a Phasic Event of Rapid Eye Movement Sleep: The Ponto-geniculo-occipital Wave." *Advances in Biochemical Psychophramocology*, Vol. 11, pp. 169 - 179.

    Knowles, J. B., et al. (1968), "Effects of Alcohol on REM Sleep." *Quarterly Journal of Studies on Alcohol*, Vol. 29, pp. 342 - 349.

    Koella, W. P. (1988), "Serotonin and Sleep." In: *Neuronal Serotonin*, Osborne, N. N. and Hamon, M. (Eds.). New York: John Wiley and Sons.

    Wyatt, R. J. (1974), "Ventricular Fluid 5-Hydroxyindoleacetic Acid Concentrations During Human Sleep." *Advances in Biochemical Psychopharmacology*, Vol. 11, pp. 193 - 197.

7. Kolta, M. G. (1989), "Effect of Long-Term Caloric Restriction on Brain Monoamines in Aging Male and Female Fischer 344 Rats." *Mechanisms of Ageing and Development* (Ireland), Vol. 48, pp. 191 - 198.

8. Wurtman, J. J. (1990), "Carbohydrate Craving: Relationship Between Carbohydrate Intake and Disorders of Mood." *Drugs*, Vol. 39 (Supp. 3), pp. 49 - 52.

    Wurtman, J. J., et al. (1987), "Fenfluramine Suppresses Snack Intake Among Carbohydrate Cravers but not Among Noncarbohydrate Cravers." *International Journal of Eating Disorders*, Vol. 6, pp. 687 - 699.

    Wurtman, J. J. and Wurtman, R. J. (1983), "Studies on the Appetite for Carbohydrates in Rats and Humans." *Journal of Psychiatric Residency,* Vol. 17, No. 2, pp. 213 - 221.

    Wurtman, J. J. (1981), "Neurotransmitter Regulation of Protein and Carbohydrate Consumption. In: Miller, S.A. (Ed.), *Nutrition and Behavior*. Philadelphia: Franklin Institute.

Wurtman, R. J. and Wurtman, J. J. (1989), "Carbohydrates and Depression." *Scientific American*, Vol. 260, pp. 68 - 75.

Wurtman, R. J. (1988), "Effects of Their Nutrient Precursors on the Synthesis and Release of Serotonin, the Catecholamines, and Acetylcholine: Implications for Behavioral Disorders." *Clinical Neurophramacology*, Vol. 11 (Supp. 1), pp. S187 - S193.

Wurtman, R. J. and Wurtman, J. J. (1988), "Do Carbohydrates Affect Food Intake Via Neurotransmitter Activity?" *Appetite*, Vol. 11 (Supp.), pp. 42 - 47.

Wurtman, R. J. and Wurtman, J. J. (1984), "Nutrients, Neurotransmitter Synthesis, and the Control of Food Intake." In: Stunkard, A. J. and Stellar, A. (Eds.), *Eating and Its Disorders*. New York: Raven Press.

9. Knowles, J. B., et al. (1968), Op. cit.

10. Friedrich, J. A. (1987), Op. cit.

11. Chaouloff, F. (1989), "Physical Exercise and Brain Monoamines: A Review." *ActaPhysiological Scandia*, Vol. 137, pp. 1 - 13.

Chaouloff, F., et al. (1989), "Physical Exercise: Evidence for Differential Consequences of Tryptophan on 5-HT Synthesis and Metabolism in Central Serotonergic Cell Bodies and Terminals." *Journal of Neural Transmission*, Vol. 78, pp. 121 - 130.

Naesh, O., et al. (1990), "Post-Exercise Platelet Activation: Aggregation and Release in Relation to Dynamic Exercise." *Clinical Physiology*, Vol. 10, No. 3, pp. 221 - 230.

Sharma, H. S., et al. (1991), "Increased Blood-Brain Barrier Permeability Following Acute Short-Term Swimming Exercise in Conscious Normotensive Young Rats." *Neuroscience Research*, Vol. 10, No. 3, pp. 211 - 221.

12. Blomstrand, E., et al. (1989), "Effect of Sustained Exercise on Plasma Amino Acid Concentrations and on 5-Hydroxytryptamine Metabolism in Six Different Brain Regions in the Rat." *Acta Physiological Scandia*, Vol. 136, pp. 473 - 481.

13. McMurray, R. G., et al. (1989), "Neuroendocrine Responses of Type A Individuals to Exercise." *Behavioral Medicine*, Vol. 15, No. 2, pp. 84 - 92.

14. Blum, I., et al. (1993), "Food Preferences, Body Weight, and Platelet-Poor Plasma Serotonin and Catecholamines." *American Journal of Clinical Nutrition*, Vol. 57, pp. 486 - 489.

15. Garrison, R. (1982) *Lysine, Tryptophan and Other Amino Acids*. New Canaan, CT: Keats Publishing.

16. Sandyk, R. and Pardeshi, R. (1990), "Pyridoxine Improves Drug-Induced Parkinsonism and Psychosis in a Schizophrenic Patient." *International Journal of Neuroscience*, Vol. 52, Nos. 3 - 4, pp. 225 - 232.

17. Haymes, E. M. (1991), "Vitamin and Mineral Supplementation to Athletes." *International Journal of Sports Nutrition*, Vol. 1, No. 2, pp. 146 - 169.

18. Bernstein, A. L. (1990), " Vitamin B-6 in Clinical Neurology." *Annals of the New York Academy of Sciences*, Vol. 585, pp. 250 - 260.

    Cowley, G., et al. (1993), "Vitamin Revolution." *Newsweek*, June 7, pp. 46 - 53.

19. Bernstein, A. L., (1990), Op. cit.

20. Cowley, G., et al. (1993), Op. cit.

21. Spring, B. (1986), "Effects of Foods and Nutrients on the Behavior of Normal Individuals." In: Wurtman, R. J. and Wurtman, J. J. (Eds.). *Nutrition and the Brain*. New York: Raven Press.

    Spring, B., et al. (1983), "Effects of Protein and Carbohydrate Meals on Mood and Performance: Interactions with Sex and Age." *Journal of Psychiatric Research*, Vol. 17, pp. 155 - 167.

    Spring, B., et al. (1980), "Psychobiological Effects of Carbohydrates." *Journal of Clinical Psychiatry*, Vol. 50 (Supp.), pp. 27 - 33.

22. Rapoport, J. L. (1983), "Effects of Dietary Substances in Children." *Journal of Psychiatric Research*, Vol. 17, pp. 187 - 191.

23. Blundell, J. E. (1992), "Serotonin and the Biology of Feeding." *American Journal of Clinical Nutrition*, Vol. 55, pp. 155S - 159S.

    Blundell, J. E. and Hill, A. J. (1987), "Nutrition, Serotonin and Appetite: Case Study in the Evolution of a Scientific Idea." *Appetite*, Vol. 8, pp. 183 - 194.

    Blundell, J. E. and Hill, A. J. (1986), "Paradoxical Effects on an Intense Sweetener (Aspartame) on Appetite." *The Lancet*, May 10, 1986, pp. 1092 - 1093.

    Wurtman, J. J., et al. (1987), Op. cit.

24. Blum, I., et al., (1993), Op. cit.

25. Engen, T. (1982), *The Perceptions of Odors*. New York: Academic Press.

26. Cain, W. S. (1988), "Olfaction." In: Atkinson, R. C., et al. (Eds.), *Stevens' Handbook of Experimental Psychology*, 2nd ed., Vol. 1. New York: John Wiley and Sons.

27. Spiller, G. A., Ed. (1984) *The Methylxanthine Beverages and Foods: Chemistry, Consumption, and Health Effects*. New York: Alan R. Liss, Inc.

28. Hirsch, A. R. (1994), "Inhalation of Odorants for Weight Reduction." *Journal of the International Association for the Study of Obesity*, Vol. 18 (Supp. 2), p. 306.

   Hirsch, A.R. (1993), "Sensory Marketing," *The International Journal of Aromatherapy*, Vol. 5, No. 1.

CHAPTER TEN: Soul Food

1. Williamson, M. (1994), *Illuminata*. New York: Random House.

   Williamson, M. (1992), *A Return to Love*. New York: Harper-Collins.

CHAPTER ELEVEN: Chocolate Cravings

1. Hetherington, M. M. and MacDiarmid, J. I. (1993), "'Chocolate Addiction': A Preliminary Study of its Description and its Relationship to Problem Eating." *Appetite*, Vol. 21, pp. 233-246.

   Rozin, P., et al. (1991), "Chocolate Craving and Liking." *Appetite*, Vol. 17, pp. 199 - 212.

   Schuman, M., et al. (1987), "Sweets, Chocolate, and Atypical Depressive Traits." *The Journal of Nervous and Mental Disease*, Vol. 175, No. 8, pp. 491 - 495.

2. Spiller, G. A., Ed. (1984), Op. cit.

3. Schuman, M., et al. (1987), Op. cit.

4. Ackerman, D. (1994) *A Natural History of love*. New York: Random House.

5. Williamson, M. (1992; 1994), Op. cit.

   Zimmer, B., et al. (1986), "Chocolate, Eating Disorders and Affective Syndromes." *Journal of Clinical Psychopharmacology*, Vol. 6, pp. 56 - 57.

6. McKean, C. M. (1972), "The Effects of High Phenylalanine Concentrations on Serotonin and Catecholamine Metabolism in the Human Brain." *Brain Research*, Vol. 47, pp. 469 - 476.

   Mosnaim, A. D. and Wolf, M. E., Eds. (1978), *Noncatechoic Phenylethylamines, Part 1: Phenylethylamine: Biological Mechanisms and Clinical Aspects*. New York: Marcel Dekker, Inc.

   Mosnaim, A. D. and Wolf, M. E., Eds. (1978) *Noncatechoic Phenylethylamines, Part 2: Phenylethanolamine, Tyramins and Octopamine*. New York: Marcel Dekker, Inc.

7. Spiller, G. A., Ed. (1984), Op. cit.

8. Poehlman, E.T. and Horton, E.S. (1989), "The Impact of Food Intake and Exercise on Energy Expenditure." *Nutrition Reviews*, Vol. 47, pp. 129 - 137.

Chapter Thirteen: Dairy Cravings

1. Logue, A. W. (1991) *The Psychology of Eating and Drinking: An Introduction* (2nd Edition). New York: W. H. Freeman and Co.

2. Kretchmer, N. (1978), "Lactose and Lactase." In: *Human Nutrition*. San Francisco: W. H. Freeman and Co.

3. Bolton, B. and Renfrow, N. E. (1979), "Personality Characteristics Associated with Aerobic Exercise in Adult Females." *Journal of Personality Assessment*, Vol. 43 (5), pp. 504 - 508.

    Dyer, J. B. and Crouch, J. G. (1988), "Effects of Running and Other Activities on Moods." *Perceptual and Motor Skills*, Vol. 67, pp. 43 - 50.

    Folkins, C. H. and Sime, W. E. (1981), "Physical Fitness Training and Mental Health." *American Psychologist*, Vol. 36, No. 4, pp. 373 - 389.

    Labbe, E. E., et al. (1988), "Effects of Consistent Aerobic Exercise on the Psychological Functioning of Women." *Perceptual and Motor Skills*, Vol. 67, pp. 919 - 925.

    Netz, Y., et al. (1988), "Pattern of Psychological Fitness as Related to Pattern of Physical Fitness Among Older Adults." *Perceptual and Motor Skills*, Vol. 67, pp. 647 - 655.

4. McCann, I. L. and Holmes, D. S. (1984), "Influence of Aerobic Exercise on Depression." *Journal of Personality and Social Psychology*, Vol. 46, No. 5, pp. 1142 - 1147.

Chapter Fourteen: Salty Snack Foods

1. Strober, M. (1984), Op. cit.

2. Rowland, N. E. and Kerr, J. (1991), "Effects of Exercise and Anion on Intake of Sodium Solutions in Syrian Hamsters." *Physiology and Behavior*, Vol. 49, pp. 1061 - 1064.

    Rowland, N. and Marques, D. M. (1980), "Stress-Induced Eating: Misrepresentation?" *Appetite*, Vol. 1, pp. 225 - 228.

    Rowland, N. E. and Antelman, S. M. (1976), "Stress-Induced Hyperphagia and Obesity in Rats: A Possible Model for Understanding Human Obesity." *Science*, Vol. 191, pp. 310 - 312.

3. Cantor, M. B., et al. (1982), "Induced Bad Habits: Adjunctive Ingestion and Grooming in Human Subjects." *Appetite*, Vol. 3, pp. 1 - 12.

Cantor, M. B. (1981), "Bad Habits: Models of Induced Ingestion in Satiated Rats and People." In: Miller, S.A. (Ed.), *Nutrition and Behavior.* Philadelphia: Franklin Institute.

4. Fray, P. J. and Robbins, T. W., "Stress-Induced Eating: Rejoinder." *Appetite,*Vol. 1, pp. 135 - 139.

Robbins, T. W. and Fray, P.J. (1980), "Stress-Induced Eating: Fact, Fiction or Misunderstanding?" *Appetite*, Vol.1, pp. 103 - 133.

Robbins, T. W. and Fray, P.J. (1980), "Stress-Induced Eating: Reply to Bolles, Rowland and Marques, and Herman and Polivy." *Appetite*, Vol. 1, pp. 231 - 239.

Rodin, J. (1980), Op. cit.

Rodin, J. (1978) In: Bray, G. A. (Ed.) *Recent Advances in Obesity Research II.* London: Newman Publishing.

5. Herman, C. P. and Polivy, J. (1980), "Stress-Induced Eating and Eating-Induced Stress (Reduction?): A Response to Robbins and Fray." *Appetite,* Vol. 1, pp. 135 - 139.

Morley, J. E. and Levine, A. S. (1981), "Endogenous Opiates and Stress-Induced Eating." *Science*, Vol. 214, pp. 1150 - 1151.

Morley, J. E. and Levine, A. S. (1980), "Stress-Induced Eating is Mediated Through Endogenous Opiates." *Science*, Vol. 209, pp. 1259 - 1261.

6. Cowart, B. J. (1989), "Relationships Between Taste and Smell Across the Adult Life Span." In: Murphy, C., et al. (Eds.), *Nutrition and the Chemical Senses in Aging: Recent Advances and Current Research Needs.* New York: Academy of Sciences.

7. Schiffman, S. S. and Warwick, Z. S. (1989), "Use of Flavor-Amplified Foods to Improve Nutritional Status in Elderly Persons." In: Murphy, C., et al. (Eds.), *Nutrition and the Chemical Senses in Aging: Recent Advances and Current Research Needs.* New York: Academy of Sciences.

8. Beauchamp, G. K. (1987a), "The Human Preference for Excess Salt." *American Scientist*, Vol. 75 (1), pp. 27 - 33.

Beauchamp, G. K., et al. (1987b), "Failure to Compensate Decreased Dietary Sodium with Increased Table Salt Usage." *Journal of the American Medical Association*, Vol. 258, pp. 3275 - 3278.

Beauchamp, G. K., et al. (1986), "Developmental Changes in Salt Acceptability in Human Infants." *Developmental Psychobiology*, Vol. 19, pp. 17 - 25.

9. Parker, H., Virtue, D. and Tienhaara, M. (1995) *If This Is Love, Why Do I Feel So Bad?* Minneapolis: Deaconess.

10. Hollis, J. (1994) *Fat and Furious: Women and Food Obsession*. New York: Ballantine Books.

11. Beauchamp, G. K. (1987 a. and b.; 1986), Op. cit.

    Shepherd, R., et al. (1989), "Limited Compensation by Table Salt for Reduced Salt within a Meal." *Appetite*, Vol. 13, pp. 193 - 200.

12. Logue, A. W. (1991), Op. cit.

    Logue, A. W. (1979), Op. cit.

CHAPTER FIFTEEN: Spicy Foods

1. Lyman, B. (1989), Op. cit.

2. Back, K. W. and Glasgow, M. (1981), "Social Networks and Psychological Condition in Diet Preferences: Gourmets and Vegetarians. *Basic and Applied Social Psychology*, Vol. 2, pp. 1 - 9.

   Kish, G. B. and Donnenwerth, G. V. (1972), "Sex Differences in the Correlates of Stimulus Seeking." *Journal of Consulting and Clinical Psychology*, Vol. 38, pp. 42 - 49.

   Otis, L. P. (1984), "Factors Influencing the Willingness to Taste Unusual Foods." *Psychological Reports*, Vol. 54, pp. 739 - 745.

   Rodin, J., et al. (1991), Op. cit.

3. Kermode, G. O. (1978), "Food Additives." In: *Human Nutrition*. San Francisco: W. H. Freeman and Co.

   Nemeroff, C. B. (1981), "Monosodium Glutamate-Induced Neurotoxicity: Review of the Literature and Call for Further Research." In: Miller, S. A. (Ed.), *Nutrition and Behavior*. Philadelphia: Franklin Institute.

4. Barinaga, M. (1990), "Amino Acids: How Much Excitement is Too Much?" *Science*, Vol. 247, pp. 20 - 22.

5. Schacter, S. (1971), "Some Extraordinary Facts About Obese Humans and Rats." *American Psychologist*, Vol. 26, pp. 129 - 144.

6. Rozin, P. (1990), "Getting to Like the Burn of Chili Pepper: Biological, Psychological and Cultural Perspectives." In: Green, B.G., et al., (Eds.), *Chemical Senses:* Vol. 2. New York: Marcel Dekker.

7. Willoughby, J. (1994), "Taste: It's Simply a Matter of, Well, Taste." *The New York Times*, December 16.

CHAPTER SIXTEEN: Liquid Cravings

1. Anderson, G. H. and Leiter, L. A. (1988), "Effects of Aspartame and Phenylalanine on Meal-Time Food Intake of Humans." *Appetite*, Vol. 11 (Supp.), pp. 48 - 53.

Blundell, J. E. (1992, 1986), Op. cit.

Brala, P.M. and Hagen, R.L. (1983), "Effects of Sweetness Perception and Caloric Value of a Preload on Short-Term Intake." *Physiology and Behavior*, Vol. 30, pp. 1 - 9.

Bruce, D. G., et al. (1987), "Cephalic Phase Metabolic Responses in Normal-Weight Adults." *Metabolism*, Vol. 36, pp. 721 - 725.

Fernstrom, J. D. (1988), "Carbohydrate Ingestion and Brain Serotonin Synthesis: Relevance to a Putative Control Loop for Regulating Carbohydrate Ingestion, and Effects of Aspartame Consumption." *Appetite*, Vol. 11 (Supp.), pp. 35 - 41.

Geiselman, P.G. (1988), "Sugar-Induced Hyperphagia: Is Hyperinsulinemia, Hypoglycemia or Any Other Factor a 'Necessary' Condition?" *Appetite*, Vol. 11 (Supp.), pp. 26 - 34.

Porikos, K. P. and Koopmans, H.S. (1988), "The Effect of Non-Nutritive Sweeteners on Body Weight in Rats." *Appetite*, Vol. 11 (Supp.), pp. 12 - 15.

Rodin, J. (1991), "Effects of Pure Sugar vs. Mixed Starch Fructose Loads on Food Intake." *Appetite*, Vol. 17, pp. 213 - 219.

Simon, C., et al. (1986), "Cephalic Phase Insulin Secretion in Relation to Food Presentation in Normal and Overweight Subjects." *Physiology and Behavior*, Vol. 36, pp. 465 - 469.

Tordoff, M.G. and Friedman, M.I. (1989), "Drinking Saccharin Increases Food Intake and Preference." *Appetite*, Vol. 12, pp. 1 - 56.

VanderWeele, D. A. (1985), "Hyperinsulinism and Feeding; Not All Sequences Lead to the Same Behavioral Outcome or Conclusions." *Appetite*, Vol. 6, pp. 47 - 52

Vasselli, J. R. (1985), "Carbohydrate Ingestion, Hypoglycemia and Obesity."*Appetite*, Vol. 6, pp. 53 - 59.

2. Anderson, G. H. (1988), Op. cit.

Fernstrom, J. D. (1988), Op. cit.

3. Virtue, D. (1991) *The Chocoholic's Dream Diet*. New York: Bantam.

Fanselow, M.S. and Birk, J. (1982), "Flavor-Flavor Associations Induce Hedonic Shifts in Taste Preferences." *Animal Learning and Behavior*, Vol. 10, 223 - 228.

4. Bolles, R. C., et al. (1981), "Conditioned Taste Preferences Based on Caloric Density." *Journal of Experimental Psychology*: *Animal Behavior Processes*,Vol. 7, pp. 59 - 69.

Zellner, D. A., et al. (1983), "Conditioned Enhancement of Human's Liking for Flavor by Pairing with Sweetness." *Learning and Motivation*, Vol. 14, pp. 338 - 350.

5. Logue, A. W. (1991), Op. cit.

6. Todorovic, V., et al. (1993), "Effects of Chronic Ethanol Administration on the Serotonin-Producing Cells." *Histology and Histopathology*, Vol. 8, No. 2, pp. 285 - 296.

7 Virtue, D., (1994), *Losing Your Pounds of Pain: Breaking the Link Between Abuse, Stress, and Overeating,* Carson, CA: Hay House.

8. Lyman, B. (1989), Op. cit.

9. McKean, C. M. (1972), Op. cit.

Mosnaim, A.D., et al. (1978), Op. cit.

CHAPTER SEVENTEEN: Nuts and Peanut Butter

1. Virtue, D. (1994) *Yo-Yo Relationships: How to Break the I-Need-A-Man Habit and Find Stability*. Minneapolis, MN: Deaconess Press.

2. Pennington, J.A.T. and Church, H. N. (1985), Op. cit.

3. Spiller, G. A. (1984), Op. cit.

CHAPTER EIGHTEEN: Breads, Rice, and Pasta

1. Marano, H. E. (1993), "Chemistry and Craving." *Psychology Today*, Vol. 26, No. 1, pp. 30 - 36

2. Hirsch, A. R. (1992), "Nostalgia: A Neuropsychiatric Understanding." *Advances in Consumer Research,* Vol. 19, pp. 390 - 395.

3. Chaouloff, F. (1989), Op. cit.

4. Dey, S., et al. (1992), "Exercise Training: Significance of Regional Alterations in Serotonin Metabolism of Rat Brain in Relation to Antidepressant Effect of Exercise." *Physiology and Behavior*, Vol. 52, No. 6, pp. 1095 - 1099.

5. Bernstein, A. L. (1990), Op. cit.

Sandyk, R. and Pardeshi, R. (1990), Op. cit.

6. Piscatella, J. C. (1991) *Controlling Your Fat Tooth*. New York: Workman Publishing.

CHAPTER NINETEEN: Cookies, Cakes, and Pies

1. Birch, L. L. (1987; 1985; 1982; 1981; 1980), Op. cit.

CHAPTER TWENTY: Candy Cravings

1. Schlundt, D. G., et al. (1993), "A Sequential Behavioral Analysis of Craving Sweets in Obese Women." *Addictive Behaviors*, Vol. 18, pp. 67 - 80.

Schlundt, D. G., et al. (1992), "The Role of Breakfast in the Treatment of Obesity: A Randomized Clinical Trial." *American Journal
of Clinical Nutrition*, Vol. 55, pp. 645 - 651.

2. Davis, C. M. (1939; 1930; 1928), Op. cit.

3. Rapoport, J. L. (1983), Op. cit.

4. Desor, J.A. and Beauchamp, G.K. (1987), "Longitudinal Changes in
Sweet Preferences in Humans." *Physiology and Behavior*, Vol. 39,
pp. 639 - 641.

   Desor, J. A., et al. (1973). "Taste in Acceptance of Sugars by Human
Infants." *Journal of Comparative and Physiological Psychology*,
Vol. 84, pp. 496 - 501.

5. Desor, J.A., et al. (1987; 1973), Op. cit.

6. Lu, H. C. (1986) *Chinese System of Food Cures: Prevention and
Remedies*. New York: Sterling Publishing Co.

7. Hirschmann, J. R. and Munter, C. H. (1995) *When Women Stop Hating Their Bodies: Freeing Yourself from Food and Weight
Obsession*. New York: Fawcett Columbine.

CHAPTER TWENTY-ONE: High-Fat Foods

1. Birch, L. L. (1987; 1985; 1982; 1981; 1980), Op. cit.

2. Bolles, R. C. (1983), "A 'Mixed' Model of Taste Preference." In:
Mellgren, R. L.(Ed.) *Animal Cognition and Behavior*. New York:
North-Holland.

   Bolles, R.C., et al. (1981), Op. cit.

   Bolles, R. C. (1980), "Stress-Induced Overeating? A Response to
Robbins and Fray." *Appetite*, Vol. 1, pp. 229 - 230.

   Booth, D.A. (1982), "How Nutritional Effects of Food Can Influence
People's Dietary Choices." In: Barker, L. M. (Ed.) *The Psychobiology of Human Food Selection*. Westport, CT: AVI Publishing.

   Booth, D.A., et al. (1982), "Starch Content of Ordinary Foods, Associated Conditions, Human Appetite and Satiation, Indexed by Intake
and Eating Pleasantness of Starch-Paired Flavours." *Appetite*, 3, pp.
163 - 184.

3. Logue, A. W. (1991), Op. cit.

4. Hay, L. L. (1988) *Heal Your Body*. Carson, CA: Hay House.

CHAPTER TWENTY-THREE: Charting Your Food Cravings

1. Hay, L. L. (1984) *You Can Heal Your Life*. Carson, CA: Hay House.

   Hay, L. L. (1988), Op. cit.

GLOSSARY OF TERMS

1. Buist, R. (1988), Op. cit.

   Coccaro, E. F. and Murphy, D. L., Eds. (1990), *Serotonin in Major Psychiatric Disorders*. Washington, D.C.: American Psychiatric Press, Inc.

   Chaitow, L. (1991), *Thorsons Guide to Amino Acids*. London: Harper-Collins.

   Garrison, R. (1982), Op cit.

   Marano, H. E. (1993), Op. cit.

   Mosnaim, A. D. (1978), Op. cit.

   Pennington, J.A.T. and Church, H. N. (1985), Op. cit.

   Spiller, G. A. (1984), Op. cit.

   Wurtman, J. and Wurtman, R., et al. (1987), Op. cit.

The following list of resources can be used to access information on a variety of issues. The addresses and telephone numbers listed are for the national headquarters; look in your local Yellow Pages under "Community Services" for resources closer to your area.

In addition to the following groups, other self-help organizations may be available in your area to assist your healing and recovery for a particular life crisis not listed here. Consult your telephone directory, call a counseling center or help line near you, or contact:

AIDS

CDC National AIDS Hotline
(800) 342-2437

Caring for Babies with AIDS
P.O. Box 35135, Los Angeles, CA 90035
(323) 931-9828
www.caring4babieswithaids.org

Children with AIDS (CWA)
Project of America
P.O. Box 23778, Tempe, AZ 85285
(800) 866-AIDS (24-hour hotline)
www.aidskids.org

Elizabeth Glaser Pediatric
AIDS Foundation
2950 31st St., #125, Santa Monica, CA
90405, (888) 499-HOPE (4673)
www.pedaids.org

The Names Project Foundation—
AIDS Memorial Quilt
P.O. Box 5552, Atlanta, GA 31107
(800) 872-6263, www.aidsquilt.org

Project Inform
205 13th St., Ste. 2001
San Francisco, CA 94103
(800) 822-7422 (treatment hotline)
(415) 558-9051 (S.F. and Intl.)
www.projectinform.org

Spanish HIV/STD/AIDS Hotline
(800) 344-7432

TTY (Hearing Impaired) AIDS Hotline
(CDC National HIV/AIDS)
(800) 243-7889

ALCOHOL ABUSE

Al-Anon Family Group Headquarters
1600 Corporate Landing Parkway
Virginia Beach, VA 23454-5617
(888) 4AL-ANON, www.al-
anon.alateen.org

Alcoholics Anonymous (AA)
General Service Office
475 Riverside Dr., 11th Floor
New York, NY 10115, (212) 870-3400
www.alcoholics-anonymous.org

Children of Alcoholics Foundation
164 W. 74th St., New York, NY 10023
(800) 359-COAF, www.coaf.org

Mothers Against Drunk Driving
(MADD)
P.O. Box 541688, Dallas, TX 75354
(800) GET-MADD (438-6233)
www.madd.org

National Association of Children
of Alcoholics (NACoA)
11426 Rockville Pike, #100

Rockville, MD 20852
(301) 468-0985, (888) 554-2627
www.nacoa.net

National Clearinghouse for Alcohol and Drug Information (NCADI)
P.O. Box 2345, Rockville, MD 20847
(800) 729-6686, www.health.org

National Council on Alcoholism and Drug Dependence (NCADD)
20 Exchange Pl., Ste. 2902
New York, NY 10005, (212) 269-7797
(800) NCA-CALL (24-hour hotline)
www.ncadd.org

Women for Sobriety
P.O. Box 618, Quakertown, PA 18951
(215) 536-8026
www.womenforsobriety.org

ALZHEIMER'S DISEASE

Alzheimer's Association
919 N. Michigan Ave., Ste. 1100
Chicago, IL 60611
(800) 272-3900, www.alz.org

Alzheimer's Disease Education and Referral Center
P.O. Box 8250, Silver Spring, MD 20907
(800) 438-4380, adear@alzheimers.org

Eldercare Locator
330 Independence Ave., SW
Washington, DC 20201
(800) 677-1116, www.eldercare.gov

CANCER

National Cancer Institute
(800) 4-CANCER, www.nci.nih.gov

CHILDREN'S ISSUES

Child Molestation

Childhelp USA/Child Abuse Hotline
15757 N. 78th St., Scottsdale, AZ 85260
(800) 422-4453, www.childhelpusa.org

Prevent Child Abuse America
200 South Michigan Ave., 17th Floor
Chicago, IL 60604, (312) 663-3520
www.preventchildabuse.org

Crisis Intervention

Girls and Boys Town National Hotline
(800) 448-3000, www.boystown.org

Children of the Night
14530 Sylvan St., Van Nuys, CA 91411
(800) 551-1300
www.childrenofthenight.org

Covenant House Hotline
(800) 999-9999, www.covenanthouse.org

Kid Save Line
(800) 543-7283, www.kidspeace.org

Youth Nineline
(referrals for parents/teens about drugs, homelessness, runaways), (800) 999-9999

Missing Children

Missing Children . . . HELP Center
410 Ware Blvd., Ste. 710, Tampa, FL
33619 • (800) USA-KIDS
www.800usakids.org

National Center for Missing & Exploited Children
699 Prince St., Alexandria, VA 22314
(800) 843-5678 (24-hour hotline)
www.missingkids.org

Children with Serious Illnesses
(fulfilling wishes):

Brass Ring Society
National Headquarters
551 E. Semoran Blvd., Ste. E-5
Fern Park, FL 32730
(407) 339-6188, (800) 666-WISH
www.worldramp.net/brassring

Make-a-Wish Foundation
3550 N. Central Ave., Ste. 300
Phoenix, AZ 85012
(800) 722-WISH (9474), www.wish.org

DEATH/GRIEVING/SUICIDE

AARP Grief and Loss Programs
(202) 434-2260, (800) 424-3410
www.aarp.org/griefandloss

Grief Recovery Institute
P.O. Box 6061-382
Sherman Oaks, CA 91413
(818) 907-9600, www.grief-recovery.com

National Hospice and Palliative Care Organization
1700 Diagonal Rd., Ste. 300
Alexandria, VA 22314
(703) 837-1500, www.nhpco.org

Parents of Murdered Children
(recovering from violent death of friend or family member)
100 E 8th St., Ste. B41
Cincinnati, OH 45202
(513) 721-5683, (888) 818-POMC
www.pomc.com

SIDS (Sudden Infant Death Syndrome) Alliance
1314 Bedford Ave., Ste. 210
Baltimore, MD 21208
(800) 221-7437, www.sidsalliance.org

Suicide Awareness Voices of Education (SAVE)
Minneapolis, MN 55424
(952) 946-7998

Suicide National Hotline
(800) 784-2433

DEBTS

Consumer Credit Counseling Service Credit Referral
(800) 388-CCCS

Debtors Anonymous
General Service Office, P.O. Box 920888
Needham, MA 02492-0009
(781) 453-2743
www.debtorsanonymous.org

DIABETES
American Diabetes Association
(800) 342-2383, www.diabetes.org

DOMESTIC VIOLENCE

National Coalition Against Domestic Violence
P.O. Box 18749, Denver, CO 80218
(303) 831-9251, www.ncadv.org

National Domestic Violence Hotline
P.O. Box 161810, Austin, TX 78716
(800) 799-SAFE (24-hour hotline)
(800) 787-3224 (TTY), www.ndvh.org

DRUG ABUSE

Cocaine Anonymous National Referral Line
(800) 347-8998

National Helpline of Phoenix House
(cocaine abuse hotline)
(800) 262-2463, (800) COCAINE
www.drughelp.org

National Institute of Drug Abuse
6001 Executive Blvd., Rm. 5213
Bethesda, MD 20892-9561
Parklawn Building
(301) 443-6245 (for information)
(800) 662-4357 (for help)
www.nida.nih.gov

World Service Office, Inc.
3740 Overland Ave., Ste. C
Los Angeles, CA 90034-6337
(310) 559-5833

EATING DISORDERS

Focus Adolescent Services: Eating Disorders
(877) 362-8727
www.focusas.com/EatingDisorders.html

Overeaters Anonymous
National Office, P.O. Box 44020
Rio Rancho, NM 87174-4020
(505) 891-2664
www.overeatersanonymous.org

GAMBLING

Gamblers Anonymous
International Service Office
P.O. Box 17173, Los Angeles, CA 90017
(213) 386-8789
www.gamblersanonymous.org

HEALTH ISSUES

American Chronic Pain Association
P.O. Box 850, Rocklin, CA 95677
(916) 632-0922, www.theacpa.org

American Holistic Health Association
P.O. Box 17400, Anaheim, CA 92817
(714) 779-6152, www.ahha.org

Office of Deepak Chopra
The Chopra Center at
La Costa Resort and Spa
2013 Costa Del Mar, Carlsbad, CA 92009
(888) 424-6772
www.chopra.com

The Fetzer Institute
9292 West KL Ave., Kalamazoo, MI
49009 • (616) 375-2000
www.fetzer.org

Hippocrates Health Institute
(A favorite annual retreat for Louise Hay)
1443 Palmdale Court
West Palm Beach, FL 33411
(800) 842-2125
www.hippocratesinst.com

Hospicelink
190 W. Brook Rd., Essex, CT 06426
(800) 331-1620

Institute for Noetic Sciences
101 San Antonio Rd., Petaluma, CA
94952 • (707) 775-3500
www.noetic.org

The Mind-Body Medical Institute
110 Francis St., Ste. 1A, Boston, MA
02215 • (617) 632-9530 (press 1)
www.mbmi.org

National Health Information Center
P.O. Box 1133, Washington, DC 20013-
1133 • (800) 336-4797
www.health.gov/NHIC

Optimum Health Institute
(Louise Hay loves this place!)
6970 Central Ave., Lemon Grove, CA
91945 • (619) 464-3346
www.optimumhealth.org

Preventive Medicine Research Institute
Dean Ornish, M.D., 900 Bridgeway, Ste. 2
Sausalito, CA 94965, (415) 332-2525
www.pmri.org

HOUSING RESOURCES

Acorn
(nonprofit network of low- and
moderate-income housing)
739 8th St., S.E., Washington, DC 20003
(202) 547-9292

IMPOTENCE

Impotence Institute of America
8201 Corporate Dr., Ste. 320
Landover, MD 20715, (800) 669-1603
www.impotenceworld.org

MENTAL HEALTH

**American Psychiatric
Association of America**
1400 "K" St. NW, Washington, DC 20005
(888) 357-7924, www.psych.org

**Anxiety Disorders
Association of America**
11900 Parklawn Dr., Ste. 100
Rockville, MD 20852, (301) 231-9350
www.adaa.org

**The Help Center of the American
Psychological Association**
(800) 964-2000, www.helping.apa.org

**The International Society
for Mental Health Online**
www.ismho.org

Knowledge Exchange Network
www.mentalhealth.org

**National Center for Post-
Traumatic Stress Disorder (PTSD)**
(802) 296-5132, www.ncptsd.org

National Alliance for the Mentally Ill
2107 Wilson Blvd., Ste. 300
Arlington, VA 22201, (800) 950-6264
www.nami.org

**National Depressive and
Manic-Depressive Association**
730 N. Franklin St., Ste. 501
Chicago, IL 60610, (800) 826-3632
www.ndmda.org

National Institute of Mental Health
6001 Executive Blvd.
Room 8184, MSC 9663
Bethesda, MD 20892
(301) 443-4513, (301) 443-8431 (TTY)
www.nimh.nih.gov

**Parents and Friends of Lesbians
and Gays (P-FLAG)**
1726 M St. NW, Ste. 400
Washington, D.C. 20036
(202) 467-8180, www.pflag.org

PET BEREAVEMENT

Bide-A-Wee Foundation
410 E. 38th St., New York, NY 10016
(212) 532-6395

Grief Recovery Hotline
(800) 445-4808

Holistic Animal Consulting Centre
29 Lyman Ave., Staten Island, NY 10305
(718) 720-5548

RAPE/SEXUAL ISSUES

**Rape, Abuse, and
Incest National Network**
(800) 656-4673, www.rainn.org

SafePlace
P.O. Box 19454, Austin, TX 78760
(512) 440-7273

**National Council on Sexual Addictions
and Compulsivity**
P.O. Box 725544, Atlanta, GA 31139
(770) 541-9912, www.ncsac.org

Sexually Transmitted Disease Referral
(800) 227-8922

SMOKING

Nicotine Anonymous World Services
419 Main St., PMB #370
Huntington Beach, CA 92648
(415) 750-0328
www.nicotine-anonymous.org

STRESS REDUCTION

**The Biofeedback
& Psychophysiology Clinic**
The Menninger Clinic
P.O. Box 829, Topeka, KS 66601-0829
(800) 351-9058, www.menninger.edu

New York Open Center
(In-depth workshops to invigorate the spirit)
83 Spring St., New York, NY 10012
(212) 219-2527
www.opencenter.org

Omega Institute
(a healing, spiritual retreat community)
150 Lake Dr., Rhinebeck, NY
12572-3212
(845) 266-4444 (info)
(800) 944-1001 (to enroll)
www.eomega.org

The Stress Reduction Clinic
Center for Mindfulness
University of Massachusetts
Medical Center, 55 Lake Ave. North
Worcester, MA 01655, (508) 856-2656